CHILDHOOD LEARNING DISABILITIES AND PRENATAL RISK

Summary Publications in the Johnson & Johnson Baby
Products Company Pediatric Round Table Series:

1. *Maternal Attachment and Mothering Disorders:*
   A Round Table
   Edited by Marshall H. Klaus, M.D.,
   Treville Leger and
   Mary Anne Trause, Ph.D.

2. *Social Responsiveness of Infants*
   Edited by Evelyn B. Thoman, Ph.D. and
   Sharland Trotter

3. *Learning Through Play*
   By Paul Chance, Ph.D.

4. *The Communication Game*
   Edited by Abigail Peterson Reilly, Ph.D.

5. *Infants At Risk: Assessment and Intervention*
   Edited by Catherine Caldwell Brown

6. *Birth, Interaction and Attachment*
   Edited by Marshall Klaus, M.D. and
   Martha Oschrin Robertson

7. *Minimizing High-Risk Parenting*
   Edited by Valerie Sasserath, Ph.D. and
   Robert A. Hoekelman, M.D.

8. *Child Health Care Communications*
   Edited by Susan M. Thornton, M.S. and
   William K. Frankenburg, M.D.

9. *Childhood Learning Disabilities and Prenatal Risk*
   Edited by Catherine Caldwell Brown

Cover: *Neonate from the nursery of the Medical Center,*
         Princeton, NJ. Classroom background from the
         Rock Brook School, Blawenburg, NJ.
Cover Photo: *Mark Hennessey*

CHILDHOOD LEARNING DISABILITIES AND PRENATAL RISK

An Interdisciplinary Data Review for
Health Care Professionals and Parents

Edited by
Catherine Caldwell Brown

Moderated by
Frederick C. Robbins, M.D.

Introduction by
Larry B. Silver, M.D.

Sponsored by

Johnson & Johnson
BABY PRODUCTS COMPANY

Library of Congress Cataloging in Publication Data
Main entry under title:

Childhood learning disabilities and prenatal risk.

(Johnson & Johnson Baby Products Company pediatric round table series; 9)

Bibliography: p.
1. Learning disabilities — Etiology — Congresses.
I. Brown, Catherine Caldwell. II. Robbins, Frederick C.,
1916-   . III. Series.
RJ496.L4C47   1983   618.92'8588   83-16284
ISBN 0-931562-11-2

To all those who suffer the hurt and bewilderment of subtle neurological differences; often devastating, seldom understood, possibly avoidable

CONTENTS

PARTICIPANTS AND OBSERVERS

Participants

Joseph Altman, Ph.D.
Professor, Department of Biological
Sciences
Purdue University
Lafayette, Indiana 47907

Sarah H. Broman, Ph.D.
Chief, Mental Retardation and
Learning Disability Section
Developmental Neurology Branch
National Institute of Neurological and
Communicative Disorders and
Stroke
Bethesda, Maryland 20205

Catherine Caldwell Brown, M.A.
Science Writer
105 Somerville Road
Ridgewood, New Jersey 07450

William L. Byrne, Ph.D.
Professor, Department of
Biochemistry
The University of Tennessee Center for
Health Sciences
Memphis, Tennessee 38163

Sarale E. Cohen, Ph.D.
Assistant Professor, Department of
Pediatrics
School of Medicine, UCLA
Los Angeles, California 90024

Don C. Creevy, M.D., FACOG
Clinical Assistant Professor
Department of Gynecology and
Obstetrics
Stanford University School of Medicine
Stanford, California 94305

Joseph S. Drage, M.D.
Chief, Developmental Neurology
Branch
National Institute of Neurological and
Communicative Disorders and
Stroke
Bethesda, Maryland 20205

Michael Lewis, Ph.D.
Professor and Chief
Institute for the Study of Child
Development
Department of Pediatrics — UMDNJ —
Rutgers Medical School
Medical Education Building CN 19
New Brunswick, New Jersey 08903

Bruce S. McEwen, Ph.D.
Professor, The Rockefeller
University
1230 York Avenue
New York, New York 10021-6399

Hugo W. Moser, M.D.
Director, The John F. Kennedy
Institute
Professor of Neurology and Pediatrics
Johns Hopkins University
Baltimore, Maryland 21205

Herbert L. Needleman, M.D.
Professor, Children's Hospital of
Pittsburgh
152 DeSoto Street
Pittsburgh, Pennsylvania 15213

Frederick C. Robbins, M.D.
President, Institute of Medicine
National Academy of Sciences
2101 Constitution Avenue, N.W.
Washington, D.C. 20418

Robert B. Rock, Jr., M.A., M.P.A.
Director of Professional Relations
Johnson & Johnson Baby Products
Company
Skillman, New Jersey 08558

Steven Sawchuk, M.D.
Chairman, Institute for Pediatric Service
Director of Medical Services
Johnson & Johnson Baby Products
Company
Skillman, New Jersey 08558

John L. Sever, M.D., Ph.D.
Chief, Infectious Diseases Branch
Intramural Research Programs
National Institute of Neurological and
    Communicative Disorders and Stroke
Bethesda, Maryland 20205

Larry B. Silver, M.D.
Deputy Director
National Institute of Mental Health
5600 Fisher's Lane
Rockville, Maryland 20857

Artemis P. Simopoulos, M.D.
Chairman, Nutrition Coordinating
    Committee
National Institutes of Health
Bethesda, Maryland 20205

Ann P. Streissguth, Ph.D.
Professor, Department of Psychiatry
    and Behavioral Sciences
University of Washington School of
    Medicine
Seattle, Washington 98105

Sumner J. Yaffe, M.D.
Director, Center for Research for
    Mothers and Children
National Institute of Child Health and
    Human Development
Bethesda, Maryland 20205

Observers

Lynne Cannon, Ph.D.
920 Highwood Street
Iowa City, Iowa 52240

Charlotte Catz, M.D.
Chief, NICHD Pregnancy and
    Perinatology
Landow Building, Room 7C09
7910 Woodmont Avenue
Bethesda, Maryland 20014

Veronika E. Grimm, Ph.D.
Director, Learning Disabilities
    Project
Weizmann Institute of Science
Center for Neuroscience and
    Behavioral Research
Rehovot, Israel

Doris B. Haire
President, American Foundation for
    Maternal and Child Health
30 Beekman Place
New York, New York 10022

Barbara McElgunn
74 Holmcrest Trail
Westhill, Ontario M1C 1V5
Canada

Audrey McMahon
2991 Princeton Pike
Lawrenceville, New Jersey 08648

Shirley Post
Executive Director, Canadian
    Institute of Child Health
410 Laurier Avenue, West Suite 803
Ottawa, Ontario K1R 7T3
Canada

Joyce Riley
406 Bay Street East
Costa Mesa, California 92627

Eleanore Rothenberg, Ph.D.
Director, Office of Health Care
    Standards and Evaluation
N.Y.C. Health and Hospitals Corp.
125 Worth Street
New York, New York 10013

John A. Wacker
10848 Strait Lane
Dallas, Texas 75229

PREFACE

When the Johnson & Johnson Baby Products Company was approached jointly by the Association for Children and Adults with Learning Disabilities (ACLD) and the University of Medicine and Dentistry of New Jersey — Rutgers Medical School Department of Pediatrics regarding sponsorship of a Pediatric Round Table on learning disabilities, there was immediate interest because of the special aspects of the proposed subject area. The subject, "Prenatal and Perinatal Factors Relevant to Learning Disabilities," was unique in that we felt there had never been a multidisciplinary review of this field and its related literature addressing subtle neurological dysfunction. We continue to feel that the impact of learning disabilities on our society commands an urgent need for prevention in terms of the number of children who turn out to be misfits or unemployed and the resulting expense to society and the taxpayer. Hopefully, there are and will be increasing means for assessment, intervention and prevention. In any event, we agreed it is essential to be able to identify the etiology of these problems in their earliest phases and then to provide a basis for preventive programs.

Sponsorship of the Round Table program included two other leading organizations: the National Institute of Neurological and Communicative Disorders and Stroke (NINCDS) and the American Foundation for Maternal and Child Health (AFMCH). Together, we set up specific Round Table objectives:

1. To collect the first specific data base on prenatal and perinatal factors associated with high risk of subtle neurological sequelae such as result in learning disabilities.
2. To assemble outstanding figures from each of twelve relevant disciplines to gain a comprehensive perspective from which to draw implications for research and prevention policies.
3. To disseminate information on possible precursors of learning disabilities for public information, professional use, and student texts.

The program outline and outstanding multidisciplinary faculty to address the broad range of its subjects were ably coordinated by Ms. Audrey McMahon, Scientific Studies Committee, ACLD, and Michael Lewis, Ph.D., Professor and Chief, Institute for the Study of Child Development, Rutgers Medical School, Department of Pediatrics. Our good fortune continued in that we were able to enlist the good offices of Frederick C. Robbins, M.D., President, Institute of Medicine, National Academy of Sciences, as moderator of the faculty's forum. Along with the rather special expertise offered by Larry B. Silver, M.D., Deputy Director, National Institute of Mental Health, Dr. Robbins provided the finely balanced national health care perspective which could only be offered by a physician/scientist in his position. We hope you will share with us and the other sponsors of this program the pride and satisfaction we feel in publishing the Round Table's summary, *CHILDHOOD LEARNING DISABILITIES AND PRENATAL RISK: An Interdisciplinary Data Review for Health Care Professionals and Parents.*

Robert B. Rock, Jr., M.A., M.P.A.
Director of Professional Relations

INTRODUCTION

As long as there have been schools, there have been children who had difficulty with learning. Slowly, these children were differentiated into groups based on known or presumed cause. Those who were mentally retarded were identified. Many others were considered emotionally disturbed. Still others were thought to have difficulty because of environmental factors. Some were felt to have not received the necessary cognitive and language stimulation early in life; others grew up in a culture that did not value learning; still others were considered the product of an inadequate school system.

Gradually, it became clear that many children who had difficulty learning had something wrong with their central nervous systems. It appeared that there was a neurological explanation for their learning difficulties. This was a dramatic turning point for education. Soon, some children who had been identified as retarded, on reassessment, were found to be of average or above intellectual potential but performing in a retarded range. Children who were considered to be emotionally disturbed were differentiated into two groups — those who had emotional problems which caused academic difficulties (the emotionally disturbed) and those whose emotional problems were a consequence of the frustrations and failures experienced because of academic difficulties (the learning disabled). Parents were no longer blamed for their child's difficulties; they were educated about their child's strengths and weaknesses and made a necessary part of the special education/mental health team. So, too, children who had been lumped together with others as socially and culturally disadvantaged or as a product of a poor school program were separated out as having neurologically based learning disabilities.

Once these children were identified it was recognized that some had difficulty with other aspects of brain function. Some were found to be hyperactive and/or distractible; some were impulsive and showed other evidence of an immature nervous system. Some perseverated or showed evidence of tactile or vestibular or proprioceptive difficulties. As different professionals studied these children, they established labels for those problems they focused on. Educators identified specific learning disabilities or used descriptive terms such as dyslexia or dysgraphia. Physicians began to label children as hyperactive or hyperkinetic, as distractible, or as having an attention deficit disorder. They pointed out other evidences of central nervous system disorder, the ''soft signs of organicity.'' Psychiatrists and other mental health professionals began to separate out emotional, family, and social problems that were a consequence of learning disabilities and not the cause of learning disabilities. There were efforts to label the total child rather than each piece of the puzzle. For example, minimal brain dysfunction, refers to a child who has learning disabilities, may be hyperactive and/or distractible, and usually has *secondary* emotional problems.

The field has come a long way. Such children can now be identified. Special educational therapy can help them learn, as can speech or occupational or other therapeutic approaches. Psychological supports for the child and family are possible.

Practically, clinically, these children are helped. But what causes learning disabilities? Can they be prevented, minimized, or even cured? If the site of the problem is the central nervous system, can basic and clinical research scientists shift their interest to this particular area and help find the answers? Millions of children each year suffer. Their interest deserve research and research funding as much as those of children with other major disorders.

This research effort has begun. Initially researchers became interested because they or a family member had learning disabilities. Later, others joined the effort because of the fascinating problems this brain-behavioral disorder posed. By studying learning disabilities one could learn more about normal brain functioning. Major efforts are now underway to stimulate more researchers to shift their work to this area and to obtain research money for work on learning disabilities.

For a body of research to advance there must be a common nosology, and testing instruments that have the reliability and validity to measure the specific criteria used in the nosology. Researcher A cannot compare his or her data with those of Researcher B unless they both agree on the criteria used for selecting children. Previous research is full of such difficulties. One team accepted children into their study because they were three years behind in subject areas; another might have accepted subjects based on a specific scatter on an intelligence test; and others were selected based on an extensive special educational battery of tests. Research on nosology and diagnostic and evaluation instruments are needed. This problem was focused on during the Round Table's forum.

Even when one can diagnose children as having learning disabilities, it is important to separate them by the course of their disability. We see children who seem to "mature" out of their disabilities by about age eight. Others show no further evidence of learning disabilities by age twelve, reflecting only the residual missing skills or knowledge from previous grades. Some will have their learning disabilities for life. Why is this true? Are there different etiologic factors that can result in the same clinical or classroom picture; can this result in different outcomes? Longitudinal research will clarify these different groups of children, each fitting under the general umbrella as learning disabled. Such differentiation is necessary for research to progress. This problem was also focused on during the forum.

Research on the brain and behavior has been slow in coming. The necessary technology had to be developed. The knowledge on neurotransmitters, the chemical messengers of the brain, led to the theory that some aspects of the problems with these children might be due to norepinephrine deficiency. Today we know of about 50 neurotransmitters. It is estimated that there might be 200. We have just begun to learn the neurochemistry of the brain.

There are other chemical activities and an expanding body of new knowledge on these activities. What controls brain behavior and interactions? Could this knowledge provide a breakthrough? Some animal research suggests a very promising lead. Research in molecular genetics begins to clarify how the genetic code results in brain development. During each phase of fetal development genetic messages result in chemicals that pass through the brain and attach to specific receptor sites in the brain, stimulating growth of that particular area. Each day different sites are stimulated in just the right sequence and for just the right period of time to result in a fully "wired" central nervous system. This process continues beyond birth and into early childhood or perhaps beyond. What is the result of a different or defective genetic pattern? Would this result in a different or dysfunctional brain? If so, could this explain the familial patterns we see? Could something interfere with these neurochemical messengers on any particular day, so that the neuronal tracks scheduled for that phase of development are not laid down? If so, what would this do to the functioning of the specific brain sites? What about the later circuitry that was to connect with these sites? Animal studies during the prenatal and perinatal period show that phenobarbital inhibits or stops this neuroendocrine process. Brain development is affected. We know little about this molecular genetic-neuroendocrine process. We must learn more. Not only might such knowledge clarify why some individuals develop brains that are "wired" differently, but it might give us a major prevention opportunity. Eighty percent of women take prescription or over-the-counter medications during their pregnancy. What do these drugs do? Could they block or inhibit brain development for an hour or a day or more, resulting in minimal or significant consequences depending on the time, amount, and length of time they circulate in the fetus? Could drugs taken during delivery or by the child during the first year of life also interfere? We do not know. We must know. We must interest skilled researchers in the study of learning disabilities.

We now have imaging technology that can study brain function while it happens. Unlike previous technology that showed brain structure, positron emission tomography (the PET scanner) and newer nuclear magnetic resonance (NMR) can show brain function. This is a fascinating and promising breakthrough. When a normal child reads, do the same areas of the brain activate and in the same sequence as when a child with a reading disability reads? Think of the many research opportunities and answers such studies could hopefully produce. But first, PET and NMR researchers must be made interested in researching learning disabilities.

We observe much about the relationship between nutrition and behavior. The research findings remain confusing. We have data on the impact of toxins (lead, mercury, etc.) and of metabolites (glucose, specific amino acids) on brain function. The specific relationships to brain functioning and to learning disabilities need to be studied.

I have mentioned but a few of the areas of exciting and promising brain-behavioral research. There are others, for example, laterality of brain functions and the developmental sequence of lateralization in each sex. There are discoveries on the scale of finding the neurotransmitters or receptor sites yet to be made. Truly, research in the neurosciences is the most rapidly advancing and most exciting of all scientific studies today.

Those of us who care about the frustrations, pain, and lost potential of children, adolescents, and adults with learning disabilities have reason to be impatient yet excited and hopeful. The knowledge base and research methodologies are falling into place. Research money is more available. More research scientists are focusing on the neurosciences than ever before. We must interest them in shifting their research interest and efforts into the area of learning disabilities. There are many competing areas of productive basic, applied, and clinical research. We must convince them that we need them — our children need them.

The joy of learning is for too many a nightmare. We can improve and improve our therapeutical remedial skills. But the real answer will be prevention. Prevention requires knowledge of cause. We have high hopes for neuroscience research.

This Round Table is a significant effort by ACLD and Rutgers University Medical School Department of Pediatrics, and the program's other sponsors, NINCDS and AFMCH, with the assistance of the Johnson & Johnson Baby Products Company to bring together scholars from many of the disciplines and fields of research described above. Perhaps more important than what was said was that they met each other, heard each other, and heard of learning disabilities and the probable relationships between their areas of research and our area of concern.

Larry B. Silver, M.D.
Deputy Director
National Institute of Mental Health

PART I

INTERDISCIPLINARY PERSPECTIVES ON LEARNING DISABILITIES

Editor's note

So many of the papers in Part I refer to data from the Collaborative Perinatal Project of the National Institute of Neurological and Communicative Disorders and Stroke (NCPP) that some background on that project is in order.* The NCPP is a large-scale multidisciplinary study of the developmental consequences of complications in pregnancy and the perinatal period. Between 1959 and 1974, children from 53,043 pregnancies were followed from gestation through eight years of age. The youngest child in the study was born in 1966.

The sample was selected to represent a wide range of pregnancy conditions and to maximize opportunities for follow-up. No attempt was made to select a sample representative of the United States population or of the communities in which data were gathered. Twelve urban medical centers contributed obstetrical patients to the NCPP. Some included all eligible women; others selected a random sample. Ninety-five percent of the women in the study were clinic patients. Thus, the socioeconomic and ethnic composition of the sample was representative of the populations qualifying for medical care at the participating institutions. Sample sizes by institution and ethnic group are shown in Table 1.

In order to assure systematic analysis of data collected in the Collaborative Perinatal Project, twenty areas of investigation have been targeted for comprehensive study. The ten primary areas are cerebral palsy; mental retardation; communicative disorders; visual abnormalities; convulsive disorders; learning disorders; minimal brain dysfunction; congenital malformations; prematurity; and neuropathology, general pathology, and placentology. The ten secondary areas are pregnancy hypertension; maternal infection during pregnancy; labor and delivery; neonatal hyperbilirubinemia; maternal anesthesia-analgesia during labor and delivery; intellectual performance at age four; physical growth; multiple births; genetic factors and socioeconomic factors; and drugs taken during pregnancy. Some of these major analyses, as well as smaller studies, have been completed and will be referred to in the papers that follow.

---

*Summarized from S. H. Broman, The Collaborative Perinatal Project: An overview. In S.A. Mednick & M. Harway (Eds.), *Longitudinal research in the United States.* New York: Praeger. In press. Used with permission.

Table 1. Sample Size by Institution and Ethnic Group in the Collaborative
Perinatal Project Population

| | **Ethnic Group** | | | | |
	White	Black	Puerto Rican	Other	Total
Institution	White	Black	Rican	Other	Total
Boston Lying-In Hospital	10,803	1,198	25	167	12,193
Providence Lying-In Hospital	2,096	672	5	49	2,822
Children's Hospital, Buffalo	2,383	59	12	15	2,469
Columbia-Presbyterian Medical Center	633	876	602	27	2,138
New York Medical College	269	1,558	2,630	17	4,474
Pennsylvania Hospital	882	8,580	316	14	9,792
Johns Hopkins Hospital	798	2,744	1	6	3,549
Medical College of Virginia	831	2,367	0	6	3,204
University of Tennessee College of Medicine	22	3,501	0	0	3,523
Charity Hospital, New Orleans	0	2,582	0	0	2,582
University of Minnesota Hospital	2,986	19	2	140	3,147
University of Oregon Medical School	2,216	861	1	72	3,150
Total	23,919	25,017	3,594	513	53,043

From: S. H. Broman. In press. The Collaborative Perinatal Project: An overview. In S. A. Mednick & M. Harway (Eds.), *Longitudinal research in the United States.* New York: Praeger. Used with permission.

GENETICS

Hugo W. Moser, M.D.

As Dr. Moser points out at the beginning of his paper, experts disagree on the exact meaning of the term "learning disabilities." In a 25-page special section devoted to definitional problems, a recent issue of the Journal of Learning Disabilities *quoted a definition formulated in 1981 by a consortium of six professional associations, including the American ACLD. It reads as follows:*

> *"Learning disabilities" is a generic term that refers to a heterogeneous group of disorders manifested by significant difficulties in the acquisition and use of listening, speaking, reading, writing, reasoning, or mathematical abilities. These disorders are intrinsic to the individual and presumed to be due to central nervous system dysfunction. Even though a learning disability may occur concomitantly with other handicapping conditions (e.g., sensory impairment, mental retardation, social and emotional disturbances) or environmental influences (e.g., cultural differences, insufficient/inappropriate instruction, psychogenic factors), it is not the direct result of those conditions or influences (Kirk & Kirk 1983).*

Even the groups that devised this definition are not fully satisfied with it. The Canadian ACLD adopted a similar but even more emphatically neurological one: "Learning disabilities are a heterogeneous group of disorders due to identifiable or inferred central nervous system damage," it begins. Other people prefer a definition emphasizing school performance (for an example, see p. 50); still others wish to stress psychological processes (see footnote, p. 87).

Although problems of definition greatly complicate the study of learning disabilities, Dr. Moser believes that progress in identifying specific disorders within this heterogeneous group can be made "by a series of successive approximations." In particular, an interplay between clinical observations and genetic pedigree analyses shows promise of being able to explain at least some types of dyslexia, which is known to occur in families.

Although it seems obvious that genetics plays some role in the development of learning disabilities, the scientific study of this matter is extremely difficult. There are three main reasons:

1. The definition of learning disabilities is a matter of controversy. The

current definition (see headnote) has value but almost surely encompasses many distinct entities. Genetic analysis requires precise delineation.

2. Learning disabilities represent a subtle malfunction of the most complex element in the human body, the central nervous system. Until recently, noninvasive techniques with which to study abnormalities in its structure and function have been in very short supply.

3. Advances in knowledge about the genetics of learning disabilities require repeated and effective interactions between diverse scientific disciplines: education, behavioral science, and biomedical science. Professionals from these fields often find it difficult to communicate, with the result that promising hypotheses may be overlooked. Interdisciplinary symposiums like the present one can help us begin to overcome these communications barriers.

Despite these problems, genetic studies need not be postponed. On the contrary, careful attention to genetic data and clinical phenomena jointly can move us toward the delineation of specific disorders by a series of successive approximations. I will illustrate this point with an example from my own field (inborn errors of metabolism), the mucopolysaccharidoses.

Genetic Analysis and Clinical Evaluation: An Interplay

The mucopolysaccharidoses (MPS) are a group of genetic disorders characterized by the abnormal accumulation of mucopolysaccharides (complex sugar compounds) in skin and subcutaneous tissues. This leads to thickening and distortion of facial features, which has caused these patients to be referred to rather cruelly as gargoyles. Mucopolysaccharides also accumulate in brain (leading to progressive mental retardation), bone (leading to short stature), and heart and blood vessels (leading to heart failure and early death).

The history of acquisition of knowledge about the mucopolysaccharidoses illustrates the constructive interplay between genetic analysis and clinical data. It is my thesis that such an approach will also bear fruit in the study of learning disabilities.

The first clinical reports about the mucopolysaccharidoses were published in 1917, when Hunter described two affected brothers in Winnipeg, and in 1919, when Hurler reported two young children in Munich. Hunter syndrome and Hurler syndrome patients (as they have since been called) resemble each other in most ways. In retrospect, however, two significant clinical differences have been identified. Hunter patients generally do not show clouding of the cornea of the eye while Hurler patients do, and Hunter patients live somewhat longer. These differences are subtle and overshadowed by the many points of similarity. It was only in combination with genetic analysis that their significance became clear.

The initial genetic studies of the mucopolysacchridoses consisted of pedigree analyses — which is where genetic studies of learning disabilities must also start. It was observed that many MPS cases showed an autosomal recessive mode of inheritance, but that in other families the mode of inheritance was X-linked. In X-linked inheritance only males are affected, while the disease is transmitted by a carrier female. In autosomal recessive disorders, men and women are affected equally and both parents are carriers.

Such differences in mode of inheritance have profound significance. X-linked inheritance means that the defective gene must be on the X chromosome. Autosomal recessive inheritance means that it must be on some chromosome *other* than the X chromosome. Thus, an X-linked and an autosomal recessive disorder cannot possibly represent the same disease entity.

When pattern of inheritance was correlated with the overall pattern of clinical manifestations, it was found that MPS patients with X-linked inheritance did not have cloudy corneas. Thus, there were at least two MPS groups: Those with sex-linked inheritance and clear corneas (Hunter), and those with autosomal recessive inheritance and cloudy corneas (Hurler).

The ''payoff'' from these distinctions came when it was found that if Hunter and Hurler skin fibroblasts were grown together, they corrected each other (Fratantoni, Hall, & Neufeld 1968). Hunter and Hurler cells thus have distinct defects. This breakthrough in our understanding of the MPS disorders has provided early leads toward specific therapies. It could not have been achieved without the earlier delineation of Hunter and Hurler syndromes as separate entities on the basis of genetic analysis and clinical observation.

Dyslexia

In this discussion, the term learning disability will be used synonymously with dyslexia or specific reading disability. There is convincing and long-standing evidence that dyslexia occurs within families (e.g., Finucci et al. 1976). Familial occurrence alone does not prove heritability, since it could be due to common environmental influences. In fact, a recent prospective study of Collaborative Perinatal Project data (Nichols & Chen 1981) highlights the importance of environmental factors in minimal brain dysfunction and learning disabilities.

There is no doubt, however, that heritability also contributes to the familial occurrence of dyslexia. Both the family studies described below and twin studies (e.g., Zerbin-Rudin 1967) support this observation. A large and significant family study was performed in Sweden on 112 families of dyslexics (Hallgren 1950). One hundred and sixty of 391 parents and siblings of dyslexics were classified as affected. In three families both parents were classified as affected; in 90, one parent was so designated; and in 19 neither was classified as affected. This pattern is compatible with an autosomal dominant mode of inheritance. In another family study, Omenn and Weber (1978) also found a pattern compatible with an autosomal dominant mode of transmission.

In accordance with universal experience, boys in the Swedish study were affected more often than girls. The repeated occurrence of father-to-son transmission ruled out X-linked inheritance. The reasons for the higher incidence of dyslexia among males are the subject of a great deal of current research. Much of it focuses on the effects of sex hormones on the developing cerebral hemispheres, as reviewed in the next paper ("Hormones and the Brain" by Bruce McEwen).

Finucci and Childs (1983) carried out a searching family study of dyslexic children. This analysis provided evidence of genetic heterogeneity. For milder cases, autosomal dominant or multifactorial modes of transmission seemed likely. However, the parental and sib status of the most severe cases suggested an autosomal recessive mode.

To sum up, the familial occurrence and the existence of genetic factors in dyslexia and learning disabilities are well established. Without division into subgroups, the pattern of inheritance of these disabilities is most compatible with an autosomal dominant mode. For uncertain reasons, the disabilities occur more frequently in males. Initial attempts to define subgroups within the dyslexic population indicate that such subgroups do exist. This supports the idea that dyslexia is heterogeneous.

Genetic Disorders

There exist a large number of genetically determined disorders in which learning disabilities may be one of the symptoms. Sometimes these disorders are hard to diagnose, so that a child classified as learning disabled may actually be suffering from an undiagnosed genetic disorder. An example is adrenoleukodystrophy, a sex-linked genetically determined disorder that first appears in boys age four to eight years (Moser et al. 1980, 1981). The most common initial symptoms are hyperactivity and school failure, and the disorder may therefore be diagnosed as a learning disability or as environmentally determined. Only later do neurological or endocrine symptoms make clear that one is dealing with a widespread progressive disorder. Fortunately, most children with learning disabilities do not have adrenoleukodystrophy or other progressive disorders, but the possibility deserves consideration from clinicians confronting children who appear to be learning disabled.

As yet unidentified specific biochemical or chromosomal abnormalities may account for the problems of some persons now classified as learning disabled without cause. Of interest in this respect are the observations of Batshaw and colleagues (1980) that persons heterozygous for genetic disorders of the urea cycle show a significant depression of verbal IQ compared to performance IQ on the Wechsler Adult Intelligence Scale. I cite this example mainly to indicate the multiplicity of causes of learning disabilities that must be considered.

New Techniques

At present there exist only three neuroanatomical studies of the pathology of learning disabilities (Drake 1968, Landau, Goldstein, & Kleffner 1960, Galaburda & Kemper 1979, Galaburda & Eidelberg 1982). These cases showed lesions in the left parietal or temporal speech region and in the thalamus. It is not known whether these abnormalities would be found in all cases. Clearly, when the opportunity arises it is important to conduct neuropathological studies of children or adults who had carefully documented learning disabilities.

A number of new and relatively noninvasive techniques have been developed in recent years. They include computer-assisted tomography (CAT scan), positron emission tomography (PET scanner), nuclear magnetic resonance (NMR), evoked response techniques, and brain electrical activity mapping (BEAM). These techniques, and other approaches that are anticipated, promise to add much to our understanding of the relation between alterations of behavior and learning and alterations in brain structure and function.

The science of genetics can make its greatest contribution to the understanding of learning disabilities when genetic analysis is combined with careful clinical evaluation, both psychological and neurophysiological. Clinical data, together with family studies, will help define the specific subgroups that make up the heterogeneous group called learning disabled children. These subgroups must be identified in order to develop specific early remedial techniques.

REFERENCES

Batshaw, M. L., Roan, Y., Jung, A. L., Rosenberg, L. A., & Brusilow, S. W. 1980. Cerebral dysfunction in asymptomatic carriers of ornithine transcarbamylase deficiency. *New England Journal of Medicine* 302:482-485.

Drake, W. E. 1968. Clinical and pathological findings in a child with a developmental learning disability. *Journal of Learning Disabilities* 1:9-25.

Finucci, J. M., Guthrie, J. J., Childs, A. L., Abbey, H., & Childs, B. 1976. The genetics of reading disability. *Annals of Human Genetics* 40:1-23.

Finucci, J. M., & Childs, B. 1983. Dyslexia: Family studies. In C. Ludlow & G. Cooper (Eds.), *Genetic aspects of speech and language disorders.* New York: Academic Press.

Fratantoni, J. C., Hall, C. W., & Neufeld, E. F. 1968. Hurler and Hunter syndrome: Mutual correction of the defect in cultured fibroblasts. *Science* 162:570-572.

Galaburda, A. M., & Kemper, T. M. 1979. Cytoarchitectonic abnormalities in developmental dyslexia: A case study. *Annals of Neurology* 6:94-100.

Galaburda, A. M., & Eidelberg, D. 1982. Symmetry and asymmetry in the human posterior thalamus. II. Thalamic lesions in a case of developmental dyslexia. *Archives of Neurology* 39:333-336.

Hallgren, B. 1950. Specific dyslexia: A clinical and genetic study. *Acta Psychiatrica et Neurologica* supplement 65.

Landau, W. M., Goldstein, R., & Kleffner, F. R. 1960. Congenital aphasia: A clinicopathologic study. *Neurology* 10:915-921.

Moser, H. W., Moser, A. B., Kawamura, N., Migeon, B., O'Neill, B. P., Fenselau, C., & Kishimoto, Y. 1980. Adrenoleukodystrophy: Studies of the phenotype, genetics and biochemistry. *Johns Hopkins Medical Journal* 147:217-224.

Moser, H. W., Moser, A. B., Frayer, K. K., Chen, W., Schulman, J. D., O'Neill, B. P., & Kishimoto, Y. 1981. Adrenoleukodystrophy: Increased plasma content of saturated very long chain fatty acids. *Neurology* 31:1241-1249.

Nichols, P. L., & Chen, T-C. 1981. *Minimal brain dysfunction: A prospective study.* Hillsdale, NJ: Erlbaum.

Omenn, G. S., & Weber, B. A. 1978. Dyslexia: Search for phenotypic and genetic heterogeneity. *American Journal of Medical Genetics* 1:333-342.

Zerbin-Rüdin, E. 1967. Was besagen die neuesten Zwillingsbefunde in der Schizoprenie forschung? *Deutsch Medizinische Wochenschrift* 92:2121-2122.

HORMONES AND THE BRAIN

Bruce S. McEwen, Ph.D.

The intimate interaction between hormones and the brain described in Dr. McEwen's paper offers a clear demonstration of why contemporary scientists have rejected the ancient distinction between "mind" and "body." The paper also shows why the more recent notion that "biological" and "environmental" influences on behavior constitute separable categories is now under challenge. Especially before birth, when brain cells are developing rapidly, abnormal hormonal secretions can have permanent effects on brain structure and function, and thus on behavior. Genetic defects can cause such abnormalities, but so can events that are environmental from the viewpoint of the fetus. Such events might include drugs taken by the mother during pregnancy, or a change in maternal hormone levels in response to severe stress.

After outlining the feedback loop formed by reciprocal interactions between brain, hormones, mood, and the environment, Dr. McEwen takes up an important and puzzling question: Why do so many more boys than girls show learning disabilities? He points out that gonadal hormones affect prenatal brain development as well as prenatal sexual development. In males, prenatal androgens appear to cause the right and left cerebral hemispheres to develop differently. Although androgens themselves do not cause learning disabilities, Dr. McEwen suggests that their differential effects on the hemispheres may increase the chances that congenital defects or brain damage will cause language deficits in boys.

The endocrine system coordinates and regulates many functions of the body and plays a key role in development before and after birth, as well as in the ongoing functions of adults. During brain development, endocrine signals can have profound effects. Timing is of the essence in the development of brain cells, and if neurons are subjected to abnormal influences from hormonal agents secreted at the wrong time or in the wrong amounts, intricate neural circuitry may be disrupted. The effects of hormones on the immature, developing brain are generally greater, and longer lasting, than those on the mature brain.

A large part of the endocrine system is directly controlled by the brain via the pituitary gland. In turn, endocrine secretions of the thyroid, adrenals, gonads, and other regulated glands act back on the brain and pituitary gland, producing a kind of feedback loop. These interactions are diagrammed in Figure 1. On the one hand, the brain controls pituitary hormone secretion. Changes in mood, as well as stressful, arousing, or joyful experiences, can alter hormone secretion. On the other hand, hormones act back on the brain to influence mood and behavior, as well as to regulate hypothalamic and pituitary hormone secretion.

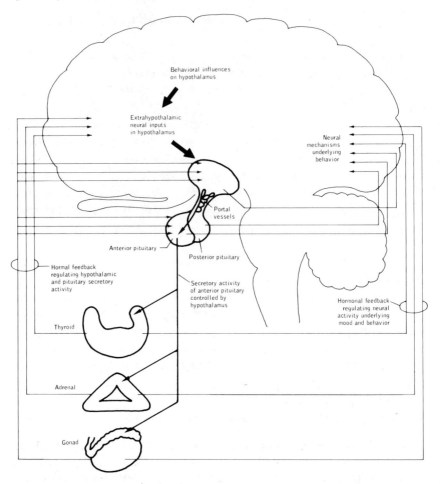

Figure 1. Feedback loop of reciprocal interactions among hypothalamic, pituitary, thyroid, adrenal, and gonadal hormones.

From B. S. McEwen, Endocrine effects on the brain and their relationship to behavior. In G. Segel et al. (Eds.), *Current topics in neuroendocrinology.* Boston: Little, Brown, 1981. Used with permission.

Endocrine alterations that influence mood and mental function may adversely affect learning ability, and they may be particularly significant in school-age children. This thesis was examined in a pioneering study of reading disability by Smith and Carrigan (1959). At that time, much less information was available than now about hormonal effects on the brain. We now recognize that besides the relatively rapid influences of current endocrine secretions on mood and mental processes, hormones can produce long-term, even permanent, effects during development by altering the growth and differentiation of neurons in the brain.

Endocrine changes that affect the developing brain can result not only from internal development programs but from changes in the external environment. For instance, separation of infant rats from their mothers leads to rapid and prolonged alterations in heart rate, arousal, and locomotor activity; it also results in rapid fall of growth hormone levels in the blood, decreasing the activity of a certain brain enzyme (Schanberg & Kuhn 1980). The syndrome of deprivation dwarfism provides a human example of an insufficiency in growth hormone in children suffering from an unstable environment and lack of a secure bond with a parent (Hofer 1981).

It is too early to tell what long-term effects such variations in growth hormone secretion may have on later brain function and behavior. Certainly, the power of environmental stress and disturbed mother-infant interaction to alter endocrine responses has potential implications for the shaping of personality and for severe disorders such as autism.

Gonadal Hormones and the Developing Brain

Many of the long-lasting influences of hormones on the brain are deduced from experiments in which fetal or newborn rodents are subjected to excesses or deficiencies of key hormones during different periods of development. Such studies have shown that imbalances of thyroid and adrenocortical hormones during brain development can have serious, long-lasting, and fairly obvious effects on adult brain function.

The influence of the gonadal hormones, in contrast, is more subtle. In male mammals, the testes secrete testosterone during a brief period of pre- or postnatal development that coincides with (in fact, triggers) sexual differentiation of the reproductive tract and brain. In rats, removal of the testes prior to this period of testosterone secretion prevents the masculine phenotype from developing; both the reproductive tract and the brain develop in a feminine direction (Feder 1981a, 1981b). The role of the ovaries in early female development is less certain. Their removal early in life does not prevent the appearance of a feminine phenotype, though certain feminine behavioral traits may be altered (McEwen 1983).

Lateralization of brain structure and function is thus linked to sexual differentiation. In our own species, the male brain is often cited as being more highly lateralized than the female brain. For example, males with left hemisphere damage show deficits on verbal tests, and those with right hemisphere damage show deficits on tests of nonverbal performance (McGlone 1980, Inglis & Lawson 1981). Brain-injured females do not show such marked laterality, though they do show deficits in test performance.

Sex Differences

As is well known, dyslexia is more common in males than in females. In addition, there is a sex difference among normal subjects in performance on verbal and spatial tasks. On the average, females score better than males on verbal tasks while males score better than females on spatial tasks.

Both these observations may be related to the greater laterality of cerebral function in males, and to androgen exposure during development. Evidence supporting this idea comes from studies of males and females with androgen abnormalities. For example, androgen-deficient males do less well than normal males on spatial tasks (Hier & Crowley 1982). Another study examined the verbal and nonverbal test performances of girls with adrenogenital syndrome, which results in partial masculinization of the genitals at birth, and of androgen-insensitive boys. Both groups had been reared as girls. The girls with adrenogenital syndrome performed less well than normal girls on certain verbal tests. The androgen-insensitive males, unlike the average normal male, did better on verbal than on nonverbal tests (Perlman 1973). These findings are consistent with the notion that androgen treatment (or presence) increases nonverbal relative to verbal performance, whereas androgen absence (or insensitivity) has the opposite effect.

Androgens and Cerebral Lateralization

What might account for the interplay between androgens and cerebral lateralization in the development of cognitive abilities? There are several theories.

According to one view, the greater specialization in males of one hemisphere (usually the right) for processing of spatial information may produce higher ability in this regard at the expense of verbal ability, which tends to be controlled by the opposite (usually left) hemisphere. This line of reasoning continues, "Strong left hemisphere specialization for verbal processing may put males at further risk for experiencing dyslexia by limiting their ability to compensate for either left hemisphere insults or unfavorable anatomic cerebral asymmetries" (Hier 1979, p. 78). The "unfavorable cerebral asymmetries" refer to situations, apparently detected in a high percentage of dyslexic children, where asymmetry of the cerebral hemispheres is reversed. In these children, the smaller and in some way inferior temporal lobe is in control of verbal processing (Hier et al. 1978, Rosenberger & Hier 1980).

Another line of investigation has noted an elevated frequency in left-handers of both autoimmune disease and developmental learning disorders. This study (Geschwind & Behan 1982) suggests that the immune disorders may be linked to the development of left-handedness and of learning defects through the action of testosterone. In male fetuses, the temporal plane of the right cerebral hemisphere usually develops earlier than the left. By 31 weeks of gestation, the left side has overtaken the right and become larger. That the left hemisphere in males matures later is further indicated because febrile convulsions during the first year of life in boys may result in damage to the left temporal lobe.

Geschwind and Behan suggest,

> Delayed growth in the left hemisphere as a result of testosterone would account for the greater frequency of left-handedness in males. When testosterone effects are more marked and neuronal migration is interfered with to a greater extent, abnormalities in the formation of the left hemisphere will result—especially in males—such as those described by Galaburda and Kemper in the left temporal speech area of a severe childhood dyslexic. This type of defect would account for the much greater incidence of learning disorders in boys (p. 5099).

In attempting to explain the mechanisms underlying testosterone action on the development of the cerebral hemispheres, Geschwind and Behan note that the neurons which will occupy the language area are formed before twenty weeks of gestation and migrate to their ultimate locations. Since twelve to twenty weeks of gestation is the period of maximum testosterone elevation in developing male fetuses (Abramovich & Rowe 1973), the hormone may affect some of these developing brain cells. It could influence their division or survival, their migration, or the formation of stable connections with other neurons. Why the result should be greater lateralization of function in the hemispheres, rather than some sort of joint influence on both hemispheres, is not known.

Indeed, explaining the possible linkage of androgens to brain lateralization is an especially intriguing problem because it presents developmental neurobiologists with the puzzle of understanding how a blood-borne substance that presumably reaches both sides of the brain can have selective effects on one side. Could it be that the hormone-receptive cells are not laid down in equal numbers on both sides of the developing brain, giving rise to an asymmetrical target for hormone action?

My own view is that androgens per se do not cause dyslexia and other developmental learning disorders that predominate in males. Rather, they alter, and perhaps restrict, cerebral development in such a way as to increase the chance that congenital defects or brain damage will have noticeable effects on cognitive ability. When we know more about the underlying mechanisms, it is conceivable that there may be ways of detecting and even preventing the abnormalities of brain development that give rise to dyslexia.

REFERENCES

Abramovich, D. R., & Rowe, P. 1973. Foetal plasma testosterone levels at mid-pregnancy and at term: Relationship to foetal sex. *Journal of Endocrinology* 56:621-622.

Feder, H. H. 1981a. Hormonal actions on the sexual differentiation of the genitalia and the gonadotropin-regulating systems. In N. T. Adler (Ed.), *Neuroendocrinology of reproduction.* New York: Plenum.

Feder, H. H. 1981b. Perinatal hormones and their role in the development of sexually dimorphic behaviors. In N. T. Adler (Ed.), *Neuroendocrinology of reproduction.* New York: Plenum.

Geschwind, N., & Behan, P. 1982. Left-handedness: Association with immune disease, migraine, and developmental learning disorder. *Proceedings of the National Academy of Sciences* 79:5097-5100.

Hier, D. B. 1979. Sex differences in hemispheric specialization: Hypothesis for the excess of dyslexia in boys. *Bulletin of the Orton Society* 29:74-83.

Hier, D. B., & Crowley, W. F. 1982. Spatial ability in androgen-deficient men. *New England Journal of Medicine* 206:1202-1205.

Hier, D. B., LeMay, M., Rosenberger, P. B., & Perlo, V. P. 1978. Developmental dyslexia. *Archives of Neurology* 35:90-92.

Hofer, M. A. 1981. Toward a developmental basis for disease predisposition: The effects of early maternal separation on brain, behavior and cardiovascular system. In H. Weiner, M. A. Hofer, & A. J. Stunkard (Eds.), *Brain, behavior and bodily disease.* New York: Raven Press.

Inglis, J., & Lawson, J. S. 1981. Sex differences in the effects of unilateral brain damage on intelligence. *Science* 212:693-695.

McEwen, B. S. 1983. Gonadal steroids influences on brain development and sexual differentiation. In R. O. Greep (Ed.), *Reproductive physiology* (Vol. IV). Baltimore: University Park Press.

McGlone, J. 1980. Sex differences in human brain asymmetry: A critical survey. *The Behavioral and Brain Sciences* 3:215-263.

Perlman, S. M. 1973. Cognitive abilities of children with hormone abnormalities: Screening by psychoeducational tests. *Journal of Learning Disabilities* 6:26-34.

Rosenberger, P. B., & Hier, D. B. 1980. Cerebral asymmetry and verbal intellectual deficits. *Annals of Neurology* 8:300-304.

Schanberg, S. M., & Kuhn, C. M. 1980. Maternal deprivation: An animal
model of psychosocial dwarfism. In E. Usdin, T. L. Sourkes, & M. B.
H. Youdim (Eds.), *Enzymes and neurotransmitters in mental disease.*
New York: Wiley.

Smith, D. E. P., & Carrigan, P. M. 1959. *The nature of reading disability.*
New York: Harcourt, Brace.

AN ANIMAL MODEL OF MINIMAL BRAIN DYSFUNCTION: MICRONEURONAL HYPOPLASIA

Joseph Altman, Ph.D.

*Before describing the studies on which his animal model of minimal brain
dysfunction is based, Dr. Altman introduces the concept of a continuum of
reproductive casualty, which was first proposed over a quarter of a century
ago but remains controversial. According to this idea, the effects of brain
damage depend on its severity. Extreme damage has extreme effects, such
as death, cerebral palsy, or epilepsy; slight damage presumably has slight
effects, such as mild retardation or learning disabilities.*

*Dr. Altman's research has led him to question the assumption that learn-
ing disabilities result from any brain damage at all. Instead, he suggests,
their source may be a retardation of brain development. Working with rats,
Dr. Altman and his colleagues have used x-irradiation at or soon after birth
to retard the development of certain cells in the cerebellum and hippocampus of the brain. The behavior of these rats on learning tasks is strikingly
similar in some ways to that of learning disabled children.*

*As background for Dr. Altman's work, two differences in the timing of
neuronal development in rats and human beings should be noted. First, the
prenatal development of the rat's nervous system takes place during a period
of only about twelve days (embryonic days 10 to 22). Second, the brain of
the newborn human infant, though by no means fully developed, is far more
mature than the brain of the newborn rat. Some neurons that develop after
birth in the rat develop before birth in the human being. Thus, the experimental manipulations that Dr. Altman and his coworkers performed on newborn
rats are hypothesized to correspond to prenatal insults to the human fetus,
or perhaps to harmful postnatal influences on the brain development of in-*

fants born early or small for date.

Learning disability is a diagnosis applied to children whose poor academic achievement and social adjustment cannot be attributed to environmental handicaps or to obvious psychobiological shortcomings such as sensory deficits or mental retardation. This diagnosis may sound straightforward. In fact, however, it rests on a controversial assumption: that the child characterized as learning disabled suffers from a dysfunction of the nervous system.

Some twenty-five years ago, Pasamanick and colleagues proposed the idea of a "continuum of reproductive casualty" resulting from different degrees of brain damage before or at the time of birth. Injury to the brain, they suggested, leads to "a gradient of injury extending from fetal and neonatal death through cerebral palsy, epilepsy, mental deficiency, and behavior disorder" (Pasamanick, Rogers, & Lilienfeld 1956, p. 617). Despite the obvious appeal of this idea, it remains controversial. Many known brain-damaged children show no signs of learning disabilities or "minimal brain dysfunction," and children characterized by the minimal brain dysfunction syndrome often show no genuine signs of any brain damage.

Hard neurological signs, the kind present for instance in cerebral palsy, are absent by definition in learning disabled children. Some children show soft neurological signs such as clumsiness, choreiform movements, and awkward gait, but these may actually reflect a mild form of cerebral palsy (Schain 1972, 1980). EEG abnormalities have been reported in a fairly high proportion of learning disabled children (Hughes & Park 1968, Capute, Niedermeyer, & Richardson 1968); however, similar "abnormalities" are also seen in children without learning disabilities (Schain 1972, Millichap 1977).

As I shall try to document, so-called minimal brain dysfunction may not in fact be caused by brain *pathology*. Evidence obtained from experimental studies with animals indicates that the learning disability syndrome can be produced by mere *retardation* of brain development in the absence of any pathology. Specifically, experimental interference with the development of brain regions in which cellular components are acquired during the perinatal period, and which are therefore particularly vulnerable during that period, can result in behavioral abnormalities in rats that are similar to those seen in learning disabled children.

Macroneurons, Mesoneurons, and Microneurons

The neurons of the nervous system may be classified into three groups, which we shall call macroneurons, mesoneurons, and microneurons (see

Figure 2). The macroneurons have long axons that connect either central nervous system and peripheral structures (such as muscles) or distant components of the central nervous system. Typically, macroneurons are large cells. They may be thought of as the superhighways of the brain.

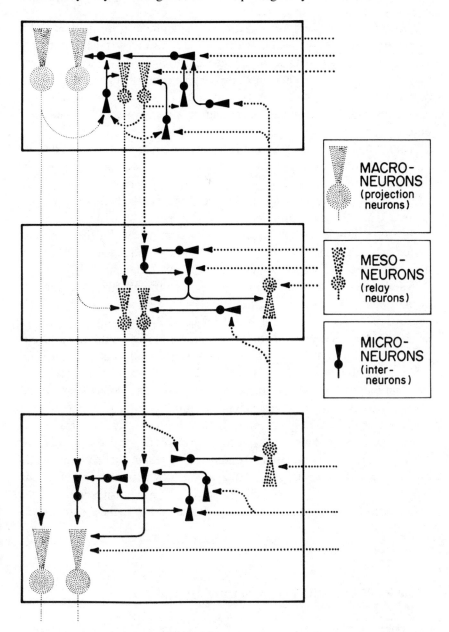

Figure 2. Schematic diagram of the interrelation of macroneurons, mesoneurons, and microneurons in three hypothetical brain structures (rectangles).

The mesoneurons connect different brain regions through a chain of relay stations where transmitted messages may be amplified, attenuated, redistributed, or otherwise modified. Some mesoneurons are large but most are of intermediate size. The mesoneurons may be thought of as the regional highways of the nervous system.

The microneurons are local elements that connect subcomponents of a single structure; they are the interneurons that contribute to the fine circuitry of a given brain region. Typically, microneurons have short axons. The cell body is either small or of intermediate size. The microneurons, which may be thought of as the country roads or city streets of the nervous system, may also be distinguished from the macroneurons and mesoneurons on the basis of developmental criteria, namely their time and sites of origin.

A number of studies have established that within several brain structures the production of macro-, meso-, and microneurons is sequential. Thus, in the cerebellum (Altman & Bayer 1978), the first cells produced are the macroneurons of the deep nuclei. The Purkinje's cells (mesoneurons) are generated next. The last produced elements are the microneurons: basket, stellate, and granule cells, the axons of which terminate within the cerebellar cortex and constitute its fine circuitry. A similar sequence occurs in the development of cells in the spinal cord (Altman & Bayer 1983).

In addition, microneurons have a different germinal source than macro- or mesoneurons. In the cerebellum, as shown in Figure 3 (A and B), the neurons of the deep nuclei and the Purkinje's cells originate in a germinal layer at the base of the cerebellum; the granule cells, in contrast, arise from the superficially located external germinal layer, as indicated in Figure 3C.

The sequential production of the three classes of cerebellar neurons, and their derivation from two germinal sources, may be a mechanism required for the orderly growth of cerebellar circuitry. The Purkinje's cells that migrate from the bottom of the cerebellum toward the surface may leave their trailing axons behind while passing the neurons of the deep nuclei (Figures 3C and D), in order to facilitate contact with the latter. The granule cells originating in the external germinal layer are known to extrude their axons in the molecular layer, where the Purkinje's cells dendrites are located, before descending past the Purkinje's cells and settling in the granular layer (Figure 3D).

Behavior of Rats with Microneuronal Hypoplasia

In our laboratory, we have studied the behavioral effects of microneuronal hypoplasia (an experimentally produced deficiency of microneurons) in the cerebellum and hippocampus of rats. Hypoplasia can be experimentally pro-

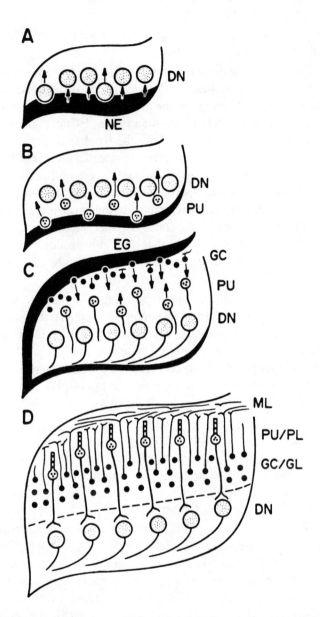

Figure 3. Major steps in the sequential generation of cerebellar nerve cells. A. Production of deep nuclei neurons (DN) in the neuroepithelium (NE) and their migration upward. B. Production of Purkinje's cells (PU) and onset of their migration. C. Migration of Purkinje's cells past the settled deep neurons; formation of a new germinal matrix, the external germinal layer (EG); production of granule cells (GC) and their downward migration. D. The establishment of the final pattern: molecular layer (ML) with the parallel fibers of granule cells; the Purkinje's layer (PL); and the granular layer (GL). The relation between migratory patterns and the apparent "spinning" of axons in the establishment of the circuitry of the cerebellum is also indicated.

duced by exposing the rat to x-irradiation after a certain proportion of the microneurons have already formed.

Studies using x-irradiation of the cerebellum at different times and on different exposure schedules indicate that severe cerebellar hypoplasia, with a reduction of over 80 percent of the granule cells, does not produce any demonstrable locomotor deficits (Altman 1976a, 1976b, Altman & Anderson 1972, 1973). In fact, in most tests the irradiated rats were slightly superior to the control rats, apparently because of a greater willingness to run after a failure. This led us to investigate the possibility that cerebellar hypoplasia leads to reduced response inhibition or hyperactivity. We found that, in young adult rats, the activity level of the experimental animals far surpassed that of the controls. We concluded that cerebellar microneuronal hypoplasia of a level of severity that does not produce demonstrable locomotor deficits does lead to hyperactivity at an age when the animals tend to be most active (Pellegrino & Altman 1979).

X-irradiation of the hippocampal region begun immediately after birth prevents the acquisition of nearly 85 percent of hippocampal granule cells, the full postnatal complement for rats (Bayer et al. 1973, Bayer & Altman 1975). Rats with hippocampal microneuronal hypoplasia are hyperactive when tested in the open field and also in running wheels (Bayer et al. 1973, Peters & Brunner 1976). In addition, irradiated rats display other behavioral changes usually associated with hippocampal damage, including learning disabilities.

Normal rats placed in a T-maze that they can freely explore tend to alternate from one arm to the other in two successive trials. This tendency is abolished in rats with hippocampal microneuronal hypoplasia. Apparently the experimental animals are either inattentive or cannot recall on the second trial which maze arm they entered before.

Rats with hippocampal hypoplasia show deficits on passive-avoidance learning tasks. According to one interpretation, this deficit reflects the experimental animals' decreased ability to inhibit an established response tendency. This interpretation is supported by the finding that experimental animals perform better than controls in an active avoidance situation in which perseveration (the animal's willingness to return to the compartment where it had previously been shocked) is an advantage.

In another investigation, Bulut (1976) used a T-shaped water maze with access to an escape ramp as the reward. Four age-groups of irradiated rats were compared on speed of acquisition of spatial and brightness discrimination tasks. The experimental animals were deficient at all ages on all tasks. The handicap of the rats with hippocampal hypoplasia was partly due to making many incorrect responses before a task was mastered. For example, a rat might adopt a spatial strategy when attention to visual cues was called for, or persevere with an initially correct solution when its reversal became necessary in order to escape from the water.

The question of whether hippocampal microneuronal hypoplasia produces memory deficits or an attentional disorder was partially resolved in a later study (Gazzara & Altman 1981). The study used a series of T-maze tasks in which tactile or visual cues in the two maze arms were graded in difficulty by decreasing the difference between them. The results, summarized in Figure 4, seem to indicate that attentional problems rather than a fundamental memory disorder underlie the poor discrimination learning performance of irradiated animals. In all tasks that were difficult or very difficult (200-300 trials to criterion for normal rats), the rats with hippocampal microneuronal hypoplasia were significantly impaired. In addition, they performed poorly on a focal visual learning task (black and white sheets were placed behind the walls of the goal arms as cues to the position of the food reward) that the control rats found easy.

HIPPOCAMPAL MICRONEURONAL HYPOPLASIA AND DISCRIMINATION LEARNING DEFICITS

SENSORY CUE	LEARNING TASK	TASK DIFFICULTY				
		Very Easy (< 75 T)	Easy (< 105 T)	Moderate (~150 T)	Difficult (~200 T)	Very Difficult (~300 T)
A. TACTILE (global)	Acquisition	smooth/coarse NO	smooth/rough NO			rough/coarse YES
	Reversal		smooth/coarse NO	smooth/rough NO		
B. VISUAL (global)	Acquistion	bright/dark NO	bright/faint NO		bright/dull YES	
	Reversal			bright/dark NO	bright/faint YES	bright/dull YES
C. VISUAL (focal)	Acquistion		black/white YES			
	Reversal				black/white YES	

Figure 4. Summary diagram of the absence (NO) or presence (YES) of deficits in rats with hippocampal microneuronal hypoplasia. The acquisition and reversal learning tasks utilized three kinds of cues (tactile, global; visual, global; and visual, focal) and five levels of difficulty, as defined by the number of trials (T) required by control rats to master the task.

In summary, the technique of focal x-irradiation makes it possible to interfere with the acquisition of the full complement of microneurons in the cerebellum or hippocampus of the rat. The behavioral effect of cerebellar microneuronal hypoplasia is hyperactivity; the effects of hippocampal microneuronal hypoplasia are both hyperactivity and learning disabilities. Thus, experimental interference with the formation of the later-generated microneurons of the brain reproduces the two most prominent features of minimal brain dysfunction in children, hyperactivity and learning disabilities related to attentional disorders.

Hypoplasia and Minimal Brain Dysfunction

No human studies provide direct evidence that the minimal brain dysfunction syndrome is associated with microneuronal hypoplasia. The few brain studies that are available have been directed at the demonstration of brain pathology. Our hypothesis is that the correlates of frank brain pathology are hard neurological symptoms and that minimal brain dysfunction is due to a reduction in the total population of late-generated microneurons without pathology.

An indirect and admittedly very weak indication of microneuronal hypoplasia (pure or impure) as a possible mechanism of minimal brain dysfunction in human beings comes from reports of its association with microcephaly. Microcephaly is common in children of malnourished or alcoholic mothers (Stoch & Smythe 1963, Robinow 1968, Quellette et al. 1977). It has been correlated with low intelligence scores (O'Connell, Feldt, & Stickler 1965), although the intelligence level of many microcephalic children is in the normal range.

Perhaps microcephaly reflects a "continuum of reproductive casualty," with the more severe cases representing impure microneuronal hypoplasia with neurological symptoms and the less severe cases representing purer microneuronal hypoplasia with minimal brain dysfunction. Support for this possibility comes from Nichols and Chen's (1981) large-scale prospective study of Collaborative Perinatal Project data. Their analysis showed that small head circumference at four months and various ages thereafter was a good predictor of learning disabilities at seven years of age. In addition, large head circumference was a good predictor of low risk for learning difficulties and hyperactivity.

The study of microneuronal hypoplasia in human beings requires a different methodology from that traditionally used in neuropathological studies. The recent introduction and development of powerful brain scanning techniques may make possible in the near future the direct assessment of the correlation between microneuronal hypoplasia and minimal brain dysfunction.

REFERENCES

Altman, J. 1976a. Experimental reorganization of the cerebellar cortex. V. Effects of early x-irradiation schedules that allow or prevent the acquisition of basket cells. *Journal of Comparative Neurology* 165:31-48.

Altman, J. 1976b. Experimental reorganization of the cerebellar cortex. VII. Effects of x-irradiation schedules that interfere with cell acquisition after stellate cells are formed. *Journal of Comparative Neurology* 165:65-76.

Altman, J., & Anderson, W. J. 1972. Experimental reorganization of the cerebellar cortex. I. Morphological effects of elimination of all microneurons with prolonged x-irradiation started at birth. *Journal of Comparative Neurology* 146:355-406.

Altman, J., & Anderson, W. J. 1973. Experimental reorganization of the cerebellar cortex. II. Effects of elimination of most microneurons with prolonged x-irradiation started at four days. *Journal of Comparative Neurology* 146:123-152.

Altman, J., & Bayer, S. A. 1978. Prenatal development of the cerebellar system in the rat. I. Cytogenesis and histogenesis of the deep nuclei and the cortex of the cerebellum. *Journal of Comparative Neurology* 179:23-48.

Altman, J., & Bayer, S. A. 1983. *Development of the spinal cord in relation to the spinal ganglia, somites, and limb buds.* Berlin: Springer (submitted).

Bayer, S. A., & Altman, J. 1975. Radiation-induced interference with postnatal hippocampal cytogenesis in rats and its long-term effects on the acquisition of neurons and glia. *Journal of Comparative Neurology* 163:1-20.

Bayer, S. A., Brunner, R. L., Hine, R., & Altman, J. 1973. Behavioural effects of interference with the postnatal acquisition of hippocampal granule cells. *Nature, New Biology* 242:222-224.

Bulut, F. G. 1976. The effects of postnatal interference with cerebellar or hippocampal development on spatial and brightness discrimination learning in infant, juvenile, young-adult, and adult rats. Ph.D. Thesis, Purdue University.

Capute, A. J., Niedermeyer, E. F. L., & Richardson, F. 1968. The electroen cephalogram in children with minimal cerebral dysfunction. *Pediatrics* 41:1104-1114.

Gazzara, R. A., & Altman, J. 1981. Early postnatal x-irradiation of the hippocampus and discrimination learning in adult rats. *Journal of Comparative and Physiological Psychology* 95:484-495.

Hughes, J. R., & Park, G. E. 1968. The EEG in dyslexia. In P. Kellaway & I. Petersen (Eds.), *Clinical electroencephalography of children.* New

York: Grune & Stratton.

Millichap, J. G. 1977. Definitions and diagnosis of minimal brain dysfunction. In J. G. Millichap (Ed.), *Learning disabilities and related disorders.* Chicago: Year Book.

Nichols, P. L., & Chen, T-C. 1981. *Minimal brain dysfunction: A prospective study.* Hillsdale, NJ: Erlbaum.

O'Connell, E. J., Feldt, R. H., & Stickler, G. B. 1965. Head circumference, mental retardation and growth failure. *Pediatrics* 36:62-66.

Pasamanick, B., Rogers, M. E., & Lilienfeld, A. M. 1956. Pregnancy experience and the development of behavior disorder in children. *American Journal of Psychiatry* 112:613-618.

Pellegrino, L. J., & Altman, J. 1979. Effects of differential interference with postnatal cerebellar neurogenesis on motor performance, activity level, and maze learning of rats. A developmental study. *Journal of Comparative and Physiological Psychology* 93:1-33.

Peters, P. J., & Brunner, R. L. 1976. Increased running wheel activity and dyadic behavior of rats with hippocampal granule cell deficits. *Behavioral Biology* 16:91-97.

Quellette, E. M., Rosett, H. L., Rosman, N. P., & Winer, L. 1977. Adverse effects on offspring of maternal alcohol abuse during pregnancy. *New England Journal of Medicine* 297:528-530.

Robinow, M. 1968. Field measurement of growth and development. In N. S. Scrimshaw & J. E. Gordon (Eds.), *Malnutrition, learning, and behavior.* Cambridge: MIT Press.

Schain, R. J. 1972. *Neurology of childhood learning disorders.* Baltimore: Williams and Wilkins.

Schain, R. J. 1980. Medical and neurological differential diagnosis. In H. E. Rie & E. D. Rie (Eds.), *Handbook of minimal brain dysfunctions.* New York: Wiley.

Stoch, M. B., & Smythe, P. M. 1963. Does undernutrition during infancy inhibit brain growth and subsequent intellectual development? *Archives of Diseases of Childhood* 38:546-552.

NUTRITION

Artemis P. Simopoulos, M.D.

Fetal malnutrition has many sources: maternal malnutrition during pregnancy, inborn errors of metabolism, and any other genetic or chromosomal abnormality that interferes with the unborn infant's ability to receive or use nutrients. Although it is now possible to identify slow-growing infants relatively early in pregnancy through the use of ultrasound, the reasons behind their slow growth rate are often far from obvious.

A common result of fetal malnutrition, whatever its source, is a newborn who is small for gestational age (SGA) even if born at term. SGA infants are known to be at risk for a variety of problems, including cognitive deficits. Dr. Simopoulos summarizes research showing that the earlier fetal growth — particularly head growth — begins to slow, the worse the prognosis for the child. These studies suggest that head circumference at birth may be the best single predictor of later development now available.

It is axiomatic that nature (genes) will not thrive (mature and reproduce) without nurture (diet). Most research on the nutritional status of pregnant women has focused on fetal growth as a measure of fetal nutrition and as a predictor of pregnancy outcome. In children with low birthweight there is an excess of behavioral and personality disorders that interfere with school performance, and an apparent relationship exists between low birthweight and learning disabilities (see ''Low Birthweight'' by Sarale Cohen). Thus, in discussing the relevance of nutrition to learning disabilities, the emphasis will be on fetal growth retardation, low birthweight, and inborn errors of metabolism.

Maternal Nutrition

The nutritional status of the mother prior to and during pregnancy is but one of the many important factors that influence fetal growth and thus birthweight. Genetic factors, placental abnormalities, toxins, the working environment, maternal obesity, various diseases and conditions, alcohol intake, and smoking in pregnancy are also known to influence birthweight and fetal outcome. The classic study partitioning birthweight variance into its components is that of Penrose (1954). He concluded that about 38 percent of the variation between different individual birthweights in surviving infants can be attributed to heredity. The remaining 62 percent, constituting the greater part of the variance, was attributable to environmental causes, including 18 percent derived from the mother's general health and nutrition.

It is generally assumed that a nutritionally excellent diet consumed by the mother during pregnancy is good for the fetus while a poor diet interferes with fetal growth. Nutritional deficits among pregnant women have been related to the greater frequencies of low birthweight infants in developing societies, whereas food supplementation before and during pregnancy increases birthweight (Lechtig et al. 1975a, 1975b). A study of babies born during the 1944-1945 famine in Holland also demonstrated that severe nutritional deprivation during the third trimester of pregnancy impairs fetal growth (Stein et al. 1975).

In a review on nutrition in pregnancy, Gibbs and Seitchik (1980) state:

> Human fetal or neonatal death or damage resulting from severe calorie and protein deficits is demonstrable from clinical experience. The impact of lesser degrees of nutritional deficit on fetal health is more difficult to identify because of the ability of the mother to provide nutrients from catabolism of her own tissues and the ability of the placenta to adapt functionally to an adverse environment.

Two recent publications by the National Research Council (1978, 1980) provide up-to-date information on the nutritional needs of the pregnant woman. The average woman in the United States gains eleven kilograms (about 24 pounds) during pregnancy. Two important factors need to be considered in giving dietary advice to an individual patient: the expectant mother's weight prior to pregnancy and the level of her physical activity, particularly in late pregnancy (Naeye & Peters 1982). Compared to women of average weight and average weight gain, lean mothers (less than 110 pounds) who gain little during pregnancy (less than ten pounds) produce excessive numbers of low birthweight infants (Niswander et al. 1969, Peckham & Christianson 1971).

Fetal Malnutrition

Any interference with the delivery of nutrients to the fetus or inability of the fetus to adapt to physiological changes that occur during pregnancy due to genetic or chromosomal abnormalities can result in fetal malnutrition. The incidence of fetal malnutrition varies from 3 to 10 percent of all live births in developed societies (Metcoff et al. 1981, Metcoff, Klein, & Nichols 1981). Many of these babies are at high risk for poor mental development. Yet, most of the mothers of these babies do not appear to be malnourished. This is because the causes of fetal malnutrition are multiple and often subtle. For example, there may be a nutrient imbalance, an abnormality in the metabolism of a vitamin, or a deficiency of a metabolite.

Fetal malnutrition may result in a newborn who is small for gestational age, even if born at term. A number of studies have been carried out on the childhood behavior of SGA infants. For example, Harvey and colleagues (1982) studied the cognitive performance of 51 SGA children at about five years of age. The results showed that children whose head growth began to slow before 26 weeks of gestation had significantly lower scores on a general cognitive index than did a matched group of control subjects. Children whose head growth began to slow later in gestation performed normally. The authors concluded that prolonged slow growth in utero affects a child's later development and abilities, particularly perceptual performance and motor ability. Lipper and colleagues (1981) investigated the determinants of neurobehavioral outcome in low birthweight infants and concluded that head circumference at birth may be the single most important variable in predicting neurobehavioral outcome.

Progress has been slow in the obstetric management of pregnancies in which the fetus is growing slowly, and few therapeutic options are available. At present, it is not known whether a growth-retarded baby is better remaining in utero for as long as possible or being delivered prematurely for better nourishment in the neonatal unit. Research is under way (using the lamb fetus as a model) to determine whether fetal nutrition can be enhanced by administering nutritive substances through the gastrointestinal tract of the fetus.

The newborn's adaptation to extrauterine life after birth requires maturation of biochemical and physiological functions during fetal development. Thus, a preterm or small-for-date infant can be expected to have different nutrient requirements than a full-weight term infant. Though beyond the scope of the present paper, these requirements are also the subject of active research and experimentation.

Inborn Errors of Metabolism

Inborn errors of metabolism in human beings, more often than not, impair development and behavior. Examples include phenylketonuria (PKU), galactosemia, maple syrup urine disease, and urea cycle enzyme deficiencies. In some cases, intrauterine nutritional therapy — giving the pregnant woman some nutrient, or withholding it — can offset the effect of a mutant allele in the fetus. In others, dietary manipulations after birth can overcome or bypass enzymatic defects. For example, phenylalanine is eliminated from the diet of children with PKU, and galactose from the diets of those with galactosemia.

Still, a relationship appears to exist between inborn errors of metabolism and difficulties in language development that may contribute to learning disabilities. Melnick and colleagues (1981) investigated the linguistic development of twelve early-treated PKU children with normal intelligence. Six children had normal linguistic development and six had linguistic delay. Data from other investigations of academic achievement and perceptual abilities also suggest that PKU children, even with normal intelligence, may be at risk for learning disabilities.

Similarly, Waisbren and colleagues (1983) studied eight early-treated children with galactosemia for speech and language function. Seven of the eight children showed deficits, particularly in the area of expressive language. Immediate recall and word retrieval skills were most notably affected. In addition, speech production (articulation) deficits were present in five of the eight children.

It is hoped that the relationship of maternal and fetal nutrition to learning disabilities will be better defined over the next decade as research enhances our understanding of the control of fetal growth and development. Research on adaptation during the neonatal period should increase our ability to minimize the handicaps and learning disabilities related to malnutrition by manipulating the postnatal diet.

REFERENCES

Gibbs, C. E., & Seitchik, J. 1980. Nutrition in pregnancy. In R. S. Goodhart & M. E. Shils (Eds.), *Modern nutrition in health and disease.* Philadelphia: Lea & Febiger.

Harvey, D., Prince, J., Bunton, J., Parkinson, C., & Campbell, S. 1982. Abilities of children who were small-for-gestational-age babies. *Pediatrics* 69:296-300.

Lechtig, A., Habicht, J., Delgado, H., Klein, R. E., Yarbrough, C., & Martorell, R. 1975a. Effects of food supplementation during pregnancy on weight. *Pediatrics* 56:508-520.

Lechtig, A., Yarbrough, C., Delgado, H., Habicht, J., Martorell, R., & Klein, R. E. 1975b. Influence of maternal nutrition on birth weight. *American Journal of Clinical Nutrition* 28:1223-1233.

Lipper, E., Kwang-sun, L., Gartner, L. M., & Grellong, B. 1981. Determinants of neurobehavioral outcome in low-birth-weight infants. *Pediatrics* 67:502-505.

Melnick, C. R., Kimberlee, K., Michaels, R. D., & Matalon, R. 1981. Linguistic development of children with phenylketonuria and normal intelligence. *Journal of Pediatrics* 98:269-272.

Metcoff, J., Costiloe, J. P., Crosby, W., Bentle, L., Seshachalam, D., Sandstead, H. H., Bodwell, C. E., Weaver, F., & McClain, P. 1981. Maternal nutrition and fetal outcome. *American Journal of Clinical Nutrition* 34:708-721 (supplement).

Metcoff, J., Klein, E. R., & Nichols, B. L. (Eds.). 1981. Nutrition of the child: Maternal nutritional status and fetal outcome. *American Journal of Clinical Nutrition* 34:653-817 (supplement).

Naeye, R. L., & Peters, E. C. 1982. Working during pregnancy: Effects on the fetus. *Pediatrics* 69:724-727.

National Research Council. 1978. *Laboratory indices of nutritional status in pregnancy.* Washington, D.C.: National Academy of Sciences.

National Research Council. 1980. *Recommended dietary allowances*, 9th ed. Washington, D.C.: National Academy of Sciences.

Niswander, K. B., Singer, J., Westphal, M. J., & Weiss, W. 1969. Weight gain during pregnancy and prepregnancy weight. *Obstetrics & Gynecology* 33:482-491.

Peckham, C. H., & Christianson, R. E. 1971. The relationship between pregnancy weight and certain obstetric factors. *American Journal of Obstetrics and Gynecology* 111:1-7.

Penrose, L. S. 1954. Some recent trends in human genetics. *Caryologia* 6:521-530 (supplement).

Stein, Z., Susser, M., Saenger, G., & Marolla, F. 1975. *Famine and human development: The Dutch hunger winter of 1944/45.* New York: Oxford University Press.

Waisbren, S. E., Norman, T. R., Schnell, R. R., & Levy, H. L. 1983. Speech and language deficits in early-treated children with galactosemia. *Journal of Pediatrics* 102:75-77.

MATERNAL INFECTIONS

John L. Sever, M.D.

Some maternal infections, such as German measles and syphylis, have long been known to cause serious neurological damage in infants before or at the time of birth. The damaging effects of others, such as herpes simplex and toxoplasmosis, are most recent discoveries. Dr. Sever reviews seven infections now known to damage the central nervous system of the embryo, fetus, or newborn. He reports that these infections probably produce a continuum of effects, ranging from miscarriage or stillbirth through blindness, deafness, and severe retardation to learning disabilities and other minor difficulties. Some infants born to mothers who have had dangerous infections during pregnancy show no effects at all.

Firmly establishing a relationship between perinatal infection and learning disabilities is extremely difficult, however, for two reasons. First, Dr. Sever says, existing studies of the effects of infections have rarely distinguished learning disabilities from similar outcomes such as mental retar-

dation. Second, infants damaged by infection are often multiply handi-capped, providing multiple sources for any difficulties they may have at school. Future research focused on specific outcomes should help overcome these problems.

A growing number of infections are now recognized as important causes of fetal damage when the disease affects the mother during pregnancy. Some of these infections can damage the developing central nervous system of the child, resulting in a variety of clinical findings such as mental retardation, learning disabilities, seizures, cerebral palsy, microcephaly, and hydroceph-aly. The damage appears to be due to direct effects of the infectious agents on the brain tissue. In most cases there is also damage to other organs.

A listing of infections known to damage the central nervous system and their frequencies in American mothers and newborns appears in Table 2. Table 3 gives the frequencies of some of these infections in a particular popu-lation: 44,000 pregnant women who took part in the Collaborative Peri-natal Project. The women were enrolled in this study from 1960 to 1966, and their children were followed in uniform fashion for seven years (Sever 1982, Sever et al. in press).

Table 2. Frequencies of Maternal and Fetal Infections
Known to Damage the Central Nervous System

Infection		Mother/10,000	Child/10,000
Viral			
Cytomegalovirus		300-2000	100-200
Rubella	Epidemic	200-400	20-40
	Non-epidemic	<10	<1
Herpes Simplex		15-150	1-5
Varicella		2-8	<1
Bacterial/Protozoal			
Syphilis		2-60	1-3
Tuberculosis		<1-8	<1
Toxoplasmosis		<1-7	1-3

Table 3. Incidence of Clinical Infections During Pregnancy in
44,000 Participants in the Collaborative Perinatal Project

	Incidence per 10,000 By Race		
Clinical Infection	White (N = 19,489)	Black (N = 20,786)	Total[a] (N = 44,016)
Rubella	35.9	28.9	32.7
Varicella-Zoster (Total)	8.2	2.4	7.7
Herpes Zoster	0.51	—	0.45
Tuberculosis	4.6	4.3	4.0
Toxoplasmosis	0.51	—	0.23

[a] Total includes all ethnic groups.

Cytomegalovirus

Cytomegaloviruses (CMV) are the most frequent cause of congenital infection in the United States. Serological surveys have shown that some one- to two-thirds of adult women have antibody to this group of closely related viruses (Sever 1962). In addition, CMV can be isolated from the cervix or urine of 3 to 5 percent of pregnant women (Hildebrant et al. 1967). Most infected women have no symptoms, though cervicitis and an illness resembling infectious mononucleosis are occasionally seen.

Congenital infection occurs in .5 to 1.5 percent of births. As many as 10 percent of these children exhibit permanent damage in the form of poor mental performance and high-tone hearing loss. Based on these figures for fetal damage and a birth rate of approximately 3.5 million in the United States, it has been estimated that some 3,500 children are damaged each year by this virus. Damage to the brain includes direct tissue destruction with mild to severe mental retardation, microcephaly, hydrocephaly, and deafness. Learning disabilities appear to be one result of this damage (Williamson et al. 1982).

A specific cytomegalovirus antibody is present in the majority of infected newborns. Infected children shed the virus for many months, and the spread of infections among family members has been well documented. The long-term results of drug therapy with CMV infants are not good. Vaccines are currently the subject of active investigation in Europe and Japan as well as in the United States (Plotkin, Farquhar, & Hornberger 1976).

Rubella

Epidemics of rubella (German measles) normally occur every six or seven years. Fortunately, with the widespread use of rubella vaccine in the United States, there have been no major epidemics since 1964. In the year following the 1964 epidemic, there were 20,000 cases of congenital rubella. At present, there are only 25 cases a year. In most of the rest of the world, however, rubella epidemics continue to occur at regular intervals.

Fetal damage from rubella can be extensive and includes significant damage to the central nervous system with mental retardation and microcephaly. Some children appear to have learning disabilities (Desmond et al. 1978). These children, however, often have multiple handicaps, including deafness, blindness, or cardiac damage requiring extensive surgery. They may also have experienced encephalitis in the newborn period.

Several states in the United States now require premarital screening for rubella antibody to determine the susceptibility of individuals to rubella. In the United States, rubella vaccine is recommended for all children at fifteen months of age. Almost 100 million doses of vaccine have now been given. Even so, approximately 15 percent of women entering the childbearing years are now susceptible to rubella—almost twice as many as prior to the 1964 epidemic. Although protection of younger children seems to have been effective in limiting the spread of the virus, it is still very important to immunize susceptible women before pregnancy. The vaccine is made from live virus and cannot be given during pregnancy.

Herpes Simplex

Herpes simplex virus (HSV) infections are caused by two strains of this virus. Type 1 (oral) produces infections in children and adults which are primarily located on the lips. Type 2 (genital) infections are usually venereally transmitted and occur primarily on the vagina, penis, or lower body. Genital HSV infections have been increasing in frequency and are now the second most common cause of venereal disease in the United States. Maternal genital infection at term is particularly dangerous, since the child may become infected during delivery and develop severe or fatal disease. Infections of the newborn are due to Type 2 virus in 90 to 95 percent of cases.

A child with neonatal infection usually appears normal at birth, but symptoms of the disease develop during the first three weeks of life. The disease is manifested in three general forms: (1) vesicular lesions of the skin or throat, sometimes with conjunctivitis, (2) central nervous system involvement, possibly with convulsions, and (3) systemic disease, such as hepatitis, jaundice, or pulmonary disease. About half the children with localized vesicular lesions have a good prognosis. The other half progress to more extensive infection. Systemic infection is fatal in over 90 percent of cases, and most survivors have permanent neurological damage.

The neurological sequelae for children infected with herpes at birth include mild to severe mental retardation, seizures, and microcephaly. Learning disabilities may be present in mildly affected children. However, this has not been well studied, and most children have evidence of multiple organ involvement.

The most feasible way of preventing neonatal herpes is to perform cesarean section if maternal genital infection is present within two weeks of delivery. In order to identify asymptomatic cases, pregnant women with prior genital herpes or a sexual partner with herpes should receive weekly virus cultures during the last month of pregnancy. Cesarean section used before or within four hours of rupture of the membranes substantially reduces the risk for infection of the child (Nahmias et al. 1975).

Varicella

Varicella (chicken pox) and herpes zoster (shingles) are caused by the same virus. In the United States about 15 percent of women of childbearing age are susceptible to varicella infection. Perhaps two percent of those infected in the first sixteen weeks of pregnancy produce children with congenital defects, including cataracts and other eye problems, brain damage, and skin scars and hypoplasia of limbs and trunk (Gershon, Kalter, & Steinberg 1976). Maternal infection just a few days before delivery is especially dangerous. It may result in severe infection of the infant, and some 10 to 30 percent of infected children die of disseminated disease. Surviving infants may show encephalitis, mental retardation, cortical atrophy, and microcephaly. Learning disabilities may be part of this syndrome, but this has not been well investigated.

Although there are tests that identify antibody in immune individuals, no vaccine for varicella is now available for general use.

Syphilis

There are 300 to 400 cases of early congenital syphilis each year in the United States. The child is at risk throughout the pregnancy. The spirochete crosses the placenta and grows in the tissues of the child. The infection can involve many tissues and cause a variety of clinical findings.

Maternal infections are reported at a frequency of about 100,000 cases a year in the United States. Symptoms vary with the stage of the illness, and patients with early syphilis generally respond well to treatment with penicillin. For the prevention of congenital syphilis, routine serological tests are used for all pregnant women in the United States. This screening identifies women who need treatment, and thus prevents congenital syphilis or at least reduces its severity.

Children with congenital syphilis or those born of mothers with syphilis who may be infected must be examined carefully and treated. The spinal fluid must be examined for evidence of abnormalities, and serological tests should be performed. Brain damage may include mental retardation and severe paresis. Some of these children appear to have learning disabilities; however, this possibility needs further investigation and distinction from other forms of brain damage. Penicillin is generally used for treatment.

Tuberculosis

Congenital tuberculosis can damage the brain, causing mental retardation and cerebral palsy. It appears that some children may have learning disabilities.

While congenital tuberculosis is quite infrequent, postnatal infection from the mother is a significant problem. Prevention requires broad public health measures including identifying and treating contacts of known cases and skin tests of high risk groups as well as immediate treatment of affected patients with appropriate antibiotics. The recent influx of people from Asia and other Third World areas to the United States has been accompanied by relatively high rates of tuberculosis and associated transmission to susceptible contacts. For this reason, physicians caring for these patients must be especially alert to the possibility of active tuberculosis.

Toxoplasmosis

Toxoplasmosis is an infection caused by a ubiquitous intracellular parasite. The infection may be either congenital or acquired, and the symptoms range from severe, generalized infection with fatal outcome to asymptomatic forms of the disease.

Congenital toxoplasmosis in infancy may be neurological, involving primarily the central nervous system, or generalized, with more widespread symptomatology. In both cases the principal findings include choreoretinitis, abnormal spinal fluid findings, anemia, seizures, and decreased mental performance. The prognosis for infants with congenital toxoplasmosis is extremely poor: Only 8 to 16 percent are normal at four years of age (Eichenwald 1957). Permanent sequelae include mental retardation and seizures, and some children appear to have learning disabilities.

Toxoplasmosis is transmitted through the ingestion of undercooked meat and exposure to cat feces, which carry the parasite. Pregnant women should avoid eating raw meat (such as steak tartare) and avoid exposure to cat feces. Infected women and children can be treated with antibiotics, but unfortunately, considerable damage may be done in infants with the congenital disease before treatment is started.

In summary, some maternal infections affect the central nervous system of the child and produce brain damage, which is seen clinically in many forms. Learning disabilities are among the defects produced by these infections. The affected children, however, are often multiply handicapped, and most studies have not distinguished children with learning difficulties from those with other forms of damage to the central nervous system. More research is needed to identify the frequencies of the specific types of neurological damage that result from perinatal infections.

REFERENCES

Desmond, M. M., Fisher, E. S., Vorderman, A. L., Schaffer, H. G., Andrew, L. P., Zion, T. E., & Catlin, F. I. 1978. The longitudinal course of congenital rubella encephalitis in nonretarded children. *Childhood Journal of Pediatrics* 93:584-591.

Eichenwald, H. F. 1957. Congenital toxoplasmosis: A study of one hundred and fifty cases. *AMA Journal of Disabled Children* 94:411.

Gershon, A. A., Kalter, Z. G., & Steinberg, S. 1976. Detection of antibody to varicella-zoster virus by immune adherence hemagglutination. *Proceedings of the Society for Experimental Biology and Medicine* 151:762.

Hildebrant, J. R., Sever, J. L., Margileth, A. M., & Gallagan, D. A. 1967. Cytomegalovirus in the normal pregnant female. *American Journal of Obstetrics and Gynecology* 98:1125.

Nahmias, A. J., Visintine, A. M., Reiner, C. B., Del Buono, I., Shore, S. H., & Starr, S. E. 1975. Herpes simplex virus infection of the fetus and newborn. In S. Krugman & A. A. Gershon (Eds.), *Infection of the fetus and newborn*. New York: A. R. Liss.

Plotkin, S. A., Farquhar, J., & Hornberger, E. 1976. Clinical trials of immunization of the Towne-125 strain of human cytomegalovirus. *Journal of Infectious Diseases* 134:470-475.

Sever, J. L. 1962. Perinatal infections affecting the developing fetus and newborn. National Institute of Child Health and Human Development Conference on the Prevention of Mental Retardation Through the Control of Infectious Diseases. Public Health Service Publication #1692.

Sever, J. L. 1982. Infections in pregnancy: Highlights from the Collaborative Perinatal Project. *Teratology* 25:227-237.

Sever, J. L., Ellenberg, J. H., Ley, A., & Edmonds, D. In press. Incidence of clinical infections in a defined population of pregnant women. Presented at the International Conference on the Prevention of Physical and Mental Congenital Defects, Strasbourg, France, October 1982.

Williamson, W. D., Desmond, M. M., LaFevers, N., Taber, L. H., Catlin, F. I., & Weaver, T. G. 1982. Symptomatic congenital cytomegalovirus: Disorders of language learning and hearing. *American Journal of Disabled Children* 136:902-905.

ENVIRONMENTAL POLLUTANTS

Herbert L. Needleman, M.D.

Dr. Needleman assumes that toxins and environmental pollutants, like perinatal infections, produce a continuum of effects in children who are exposed to them. That is, if a high dose of a substance is toxic, a low dose probably is too, though its effects may be less dramatic and less obvious. To support this assumption, Dr. Needleman describes findings from his laboratory concerning the school performance of children exposed to low levels of lead. These children showed deficits in IQ, attention, and other behaviors related to learning disabilities.

In addition, the history of the scientific understanding of lead poisoning reveals a steady decline in the level of lead exposure thought to be dangerous. Dr. Needleman reviews this history, and concludes by suggesting several other chemicals whose prenatal effects should be studied in detail.

Of the many industrial chemicals that find their way into the environment, a substantial number are demonstrated neurotoxins at high doses. It is reasonable to ask which of these agents can pass through the maternal placenta and reach the developing gamete, embryo, or fetus, and with what effects. Altered behavior on the part of the developing child is one possible result of neurotoxicity at lesser doses.

Discovery of the effects of an environmental toxin is relatively easy when the agent expresses itself in immediate, dramatic ways. But when toxic effects are less dramatic, or occur after a period of time, the harmful potential of the chemical may evade discovery. Had thalidomide caused learning disabilities instead of limb deformities, it might still be in use today.

Human knowledge of the adverse effects of a given chemical upon health generally follows a typical history. The toxicity of the agent is first recognized when workers, who experience the highest exposures, become ill. The effects on individuals in the surrounding community are noticed next, often after accidental spills or ventings. With more sensitive methods of evaluation and more rigorous epidemiologic investigations, the threshold for adverse effects undergoes downward revision. New expressions of toxicity are recognized, and the definition of the toxic syndrome is broadened. This history is exemplified by our understanding of lead, the oldest and best studied neurotoxin.

Lead

Descriptions of lead toxicity reach back into antiquity. The Hellenic Greeks provided accurate descriptions of its hazards, and Pliny warned of breathing the fumes of lead during smelting. Benjamin Franklin wrote of the effects of lead on the health of tinkers, painters, and smelters. At about the same time, the Devonshire colic, a community epidemic in England, was studied by Sir George Baker, and the cause, lead used in the making of cider, established.

The dire effects of lead exposure for both male and female factory workers was recognized by British factory inspectors at the turn of the century. Women who worked in the pottery industry were likely to be barren, or their offspring stillborn. Those infants born alive had an extraordinarily high death rate in the first year and were at high risk for macrocephaly.

In the early part of the twentieth century, attention shifted from industrial to childhood lead exposure. Ingestion of paint was believed to be the major source of high-dose lead (Lin-Fu 1980). In the early 1970s, studies of children living near lead smelters showed a troubling prevalence of elevated blood lead levels, and one study showed a lead-associated deficit in IQ.

Some studies of children suggest that lead doses below those that produce stark symptoms still induce changes in neuropsychologic function (Baloh, Sturm, & Green 1975, de la Burde & Choate 1974, Landrigan et al. 1975, McNeil & Ptasnik 1975, Perino & Ernhart 1974). My own group has studied the effects of low doses of lead by examining a large number of children considered asymptomatic for lead (Needleman et al. 1979). We measured the level of lead in their teeth. When children with elevated dentine lead levels were compared to others (controlling for 39 other variables), significant lead-related deficits in IQ, speech processing, attention, and classroom behavior were observed. Figure 5 shows the percentage of children receiving negative ratings from teachers on eleven classroom behaviors. A clear dose relationship is seen. Figure 6 shows the cumulative frequency distribution of verbal IQ scores in high and low lead subjects. A fourfold increase in IQ scores below 80 is seen in high lead subjects (Needleman, Leviton, & Bellinger 1982).

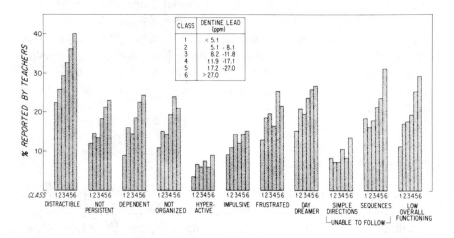

Figure 5. Teachers' ratings of children exposed to low levels of lead on eleven classroom behaviors. The children with the largest amounts of lead in their teeth (Class 6) received the highest number of negative ratings; those with the least (Class 1), the fewest negative ratings.

Reprinted with permission from the *New England Journal of Medicine* 300:689-695, 1979.

As it became increasingly clear that the threshold for lead toxicity was much lower than had previously been thought and that younger organisms were highly sensitive to lead, scientific attention shifted to the hazards of prenatal, even preconceptual, exposure. Studies in Glasgow, where high levels of lead in drinking water are common, showed that pregnant women who lived in homes where the water was leaded were almost twice as likely as others to bear retarded offspring. Blood lead levels of week-old retarded infants, obtained from PKU screening samples, showed significantly higher lead levels than normal controls (Moore, Meredith, & Goldberg 1977).

Lead crosses the placenta, and its concentration in cord blood is correlated with maternal levels. A recent study of 4,000 infants indicated that maternal lead exposure was associated with increased risk for minor congenital anomaly (Needleman, Rabinowitz, & Leviton 1983).

The story of lead may be paralleled by other chemicals that possess neurotoxic, mutagenic, or teratogenic properties. The remainder of this

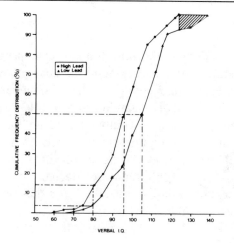

Figure 6. Cumulative frequency distribution of verbal IQ scores in high and low lead subjects.

paper will suggest several candidates (though there are many more) that are worthy of intensive laboratory and epidemiologic investigation: cadmium, methylmercury, and estrogen-like substances.

Cadmium

One is struck, upon reviewing the literature on cadmium, with the similarity of its effects to those of lead. Like lead, cadmium produces renal tubular damage, alters myocardial irritability, inhibits spermatogenesis, and damages the central nervous system (Mennear 1979). Cadmium can produce CNS hemorrhages in the newborn rat, and affects spinal sensory ganglia in older animals. It readily penetrates the blood-brain barrier in fetal rats (Lucis, Lucis, & Shaikh 1972). At relatively low concentrations, cadmium inhibits the outgrowth of cultured cerebellar cells, alters brain levels of neurotransmitters, and affects spontaneous motor activity (Singhal & Merali 1980).

Although teratologic effects of cadmium have been shown in a number of animal species, the literature on human behavioral effects is sparse. In one study, a large number of trace elements in the hair of learning disabled children were compared with elements in the hair of normal controls (Pihl & Parkes 1977). The investigators reported that cadmium, manganese, and lithium predicted learning dysfunction in a discriminant analysis model with 98 percent accuracy. However, lead was highly correlated with cadmium in this study and could not be entered into the model separately.

Methylmercury

Methylmercury is perhaps the most dramatic example of a teratogenic metal. The well-known Minamata epidemic in Japan called attention to its severe neurotoxic and teratogenic properties. Infants exposed in utero through maternal ingestion of contaminated fish suffered severe intellectual and motor damage. The largest outbreak of methylmercury poisoning occurred in Iraq in 1971. Iraqi farmers given seed grain treated with an organic mercurial fungicide baked the grain into bread instead of planting it. Thousands of adults and children were affected.

Whether mercury affects the brain at doses below those found in these two epidemics has not been studied, but the possibility should be investigated. The presence of alkylated mercury in marine life suggests that human exposure to the metal may be widespread.

Estrogen-like Substances

The responsiveness of the developing nervous system to gonadal hormones has been dealt with elsewhere in this volume (see ''Hormones and the Brain'' by Bruce McEwen). It deserves emphasis that many compounds not labeled as containing hormones possess estrogenic properties, including some pesticides. Some naturally occurring fungi are estrogenic, and the use of estrogenic substances to fatten cattle presents another route for human exposure. The impact of exposure during the embryonic period of cell specialization is a subject for uneasy conjecture.

Future Studies

Most epidemiological studies of chemical teratogens have been surveillance programs designed to detect changes in the incidence of anomalies. Investigations of this type are essential public health activities. Testing causal hypotheses, however, requires carefully controlled research. Among the outcomes that should be evaluated are fertility, fetal death, congenital anomalies, intrauterine growth, and central nervous system function. Because not all effects are evident at birth, a longitudinal design should be employed to follow infants forward in time.

The belief that unborn infants are protected by nature and the placenta from the vicissitudes of life dies hard. We know now that the period of rapid cell growth and specialization is a time of increased vulnerability to nutritional shortage and toxic excess. The need for rigorous research to identify toxic chemicals and the risks associated with them is clear. It seems equally clear that a prudent society will not await unimpeachable proof before removing these agents from the proximity of its children.

REFERENCES

Baloh, R., Sturm, R., & Green, B. 1975. Neuropsychological effects of chronic asymptomatic increased lead absorption. *Archives of Neurology* 32:326-330.

de la Burde, B., & Choate, M. S. 1974. Early asymptomatic lead exposure and development at school age. *Journal of Pediatrics* 87:638-642.

Lin-Fu, J. 1980. Lead poisoning and undue lead exposure in children: History and current status. In H. L. Needleman (Ed.), *Low level lead exposure: The clinical implications of current research.* New York: Raven Press.

Landrigan, P. J., Whitworth, R. H., Baloh, R. W., Staehling, N. W., Barthel, W. F., & Rosenblum, B. F. 1975. Neuropsychological dysfunction in children with chronic low level lead exposure. *Lancet* 1:708-712.

Lucis, O. J., Lucis, R., & Shaikh, Z. A. 1972. Cadmium in pregnancy and lactation. *Archives of Environmental Health* 25:14-22.

McNeil, J. L., & Ptasnik, J. S. 1975. Epidemiological study of a lead contaminated area. Draft, final report, International Lead-Zinc Research Organization.

Mennear, J. H. 1979. *Cadmium toxicity.* New York: Marcel Dekker.

Moore, M. R., Meredith, P. A., & Goldberg, A. 1977. A retrospective analysis of blood lead in mentally retarded children. *Lancet* 1:717-719.

Needleman, H. L., Gunnoe, C. G., Leviton, A., Reed, R., Peresie, H., Maher, C., & Barrett, P. 1979. Deficits in psychologic and classroom performance of children with elevated dentine lead levels. *New England Journal of Medicine* 300:689-695.

Needleman, H. L., Leviton, A., & Bellinger, D. 1982. Lead-associated intellectual deficit. *New England Journal of Medicine* 306:367.

Needleman, H. L., Rabinowitz, M. B., & Leviton, A. 1983. The risk of minor congenital anomalies in relation to umbilical cord blood lead levels. *Pediatric Research* 17:300A.

Perino, J., & Ernhart, C. B. 1974. The relationship of subclinical lead level to cognitive sensorimotor impairment in black preschoolers. *Journal of Learning Disabilities* 7:616-620.

Pihl, R. O., & Parkes, M. 1977. Hair element content in learning disabled children. *Science* 198:204-206.

Singhal, R. Z., & Merali, Z. 1980. Biochemical toxicity of cadmium. In J. Mennear (Ed.), *Cadmium toxicity.* New York: Marcel Dekker.

PRENATAL DRUGS

David B. Gray, Ph.D.
and Sumner J. Yaffe, M. D.

Almost all pregnant women take some drug during pregnancy, and most take several (often on the advice of their physicians). Both multiple drug use and the difficulty of finding a drug-free control group create problems for researchers who wish to study the effects of a particular drug on the fetus or child.

Drs. Gray and Yaffe describe two approaches to research on one drug often prescribed for use during pregnancy, phenobarbital. The first approach is epidemiological; research of this type indicates a slight increase in the risk for learning disabilities in children whose mothers took barbiturates during pregnancy. The second approach is experimental. It shows that phenobarbital damages the central nervous systems and endocrine systems of rodents exposed to it before and after birth, and that the drug also causes abnormalities in learned and unlearned behavior. Additional research of both types is needed not only to refine our understanding of phenobarbital effects but to evaluate the many other drugs whose effects on the developing fetus are unknown.

Pregnancy is a period of excitement, expectation, and stress. The desire of the expectant mother to provide good care for her developing fetus and to remain healthy herself brings her into close contact with health care professionals. As a consequence of these frequent interactions, the probability of drugs being prescribed for the treatment of the mother's physical and emotional problems increases. However, the overwhelming majority of prescription and nonprescription drugs have not been tested for possible teratogenic effects on the developing fetus. In some instances, the best medical care for the mother may result in serious morphological and behavioral abnormalities as the fetus develops into a mature adult. This paradox of modern medicine requires investigation.

An examination of Collaborative Perinatal Project data by Heinonen and colleagues (1977) revealed that more than 2,000 specific drugs were taken by the 53,000 study participants during pregnancy. The investigators classified the active ingredients in these drugs into 45 categories. Fewer than 6 percent of the women reported taking no drugs during pregnancy, and the mean number of different preparations taken was just under four.

The purpose of this report is to present two current approaches to the study of drug use during pregnancy. Both strategies will focus on one drug, phenobarbital, though they can and have been used to study many other drugs as well. Phenobarbital has been singled out largely because of the frequency of its use. Epidemiological studies indicate that many pregnant women took barbiturates during the 1950s and 1960s. Although barbiturates have been prescribed less frequently in the 1970s and 1980s, phenobarbital continues to be used in 10 percent of all pregnancies (Reinisch & Sanders 1982).

Phenobarbital: Epidemiological Findings

In a major study using Collaborative Perinatal Project data, Nichols and Chen (1981) identified children with learning difficulties based on psychological examinations of some 30,000 children at age seven. Excluded from the cohort were children with IQs under 80 and those with clear neurological abnormalities. Table 4 shows the ten most frequently reported categories of drugs used by the mothers of the children in the cohort (Nichols, personal communication 1983). As indicated there, 27 percent of these mothers reported using barbiturates at some time during pregnancy. Their children were found to have a 13 percent increase in the risk of learning difficulties. A small increase in risk can be important in terms of the number of children affected when both the condition and the risk factor are common, as in this case.

A problem with epidemiological findings is that correlation does not imply causation. The conditions for which a drug is prescribed are confounding variables that may affect outcomes. Additional multivariate studies focusing on specific drugs and the specific conditions for which they are taken are needed to refine correlational analyses.

Experimental Findings: CNS and Hormones

Over the past several decades, animal models have been used to examine the influence of phenobarbital (PB) on the development of the central nervous system, endocrine system, and sexual dimorphism. Several studies have shown that the brains of mice and rats treated with PB during early development weigh less than those of controls and show significant deficits in neural growth. Pre- and postnatal exposure to PB decreases total brain weight, cerebellar tissue weight, and cerebral tissue weight by about 8 to 12 percent in both sexes of rats and mice (Diaz, Schain, & Bailey 1977, Yanai & Bergman 1981).

Pre- and postnatal administration of phenobarbital can have a detrimental effect on the biochemistry of the brain (Manning, Stout, & Zemp 1971, Zemp & Middaugh 1975, Middaugh et al. 1981). It can also affect hormone levels and consequently, sexual differentiation. Male rats exposed to PB dur-

Table 4. Ten Categories of Drugs Reported Used Most Frequently During Pregnancy by the Mothers of 28,345 Collaborative Perinatal Project Children

Drug Category	Number and Percent Using Drug
Nonaddicting analgesics and antipyretics	20,206 (71%)
Immunizing agents	13,280 (47%)
Diuretics	9,480 (33%)
Caffeine and other Xanthine derivatives	8,427 (30%)
Antihistamines and antinauseants	8,116 (29%)
Barbiturates	7,730 (27%)
Sympathomimetic drugs	6,515 (23%)
Antibiotics	5,646 (20%)
Narcotic analgesics	4,185 (15%)
Expectorants	3,950 (14%)

Data provided by Dr. Paul L. Nichols, National Institute of Neurological and Communicative Disorders and Stroke, National Institute of Health.

ing gestation showed a marked decrease in testicular synthesis of testosterone on the day of birth, and the level of testosterone remained low throughout adult life (Gupta, Shapiro, & Yaffe in press). When PB is given in high enough doses, male sexual, and probably brain, development is irreversibly altered (Clemens, Popham, & Ruppert 1979). Female offspring also show pervasive hormonal effects. The onset of puberty is delayed; the estrous cycle is disrupted; and there are more infertile females (Gupta, Sonawane, & Yaffe 1980).

Experimental Findings: Behavior

A wide variety of tests have been used to assess the effects of early exposure to phenobarbital on the learned and unlearned behavior of animals. One finding of such tests is that when PB is administered during the last trimester of pregnancy—at which time the nervous system of the rat fetus is considerably less mature than that of the human fetus—the development of motor reflexes in offspring is delayed (Middaugh et al. 1972). In addition, recent studies of prenatal PB exposure indicate an increased general activity level after birth. Male rats exposed to PB during the last trimester of gestation, tested 75 days after birth, showed a significantly higher level of open field activity than untreated controls (Middaugh, Santos, & Zemp 1975a). Postnatal administration of PB to rats also leads to high activity in open field tests (Diaz et al. 1977). Interestingly, the same dose administered at the same time results in high activity levels for male offspring but not for females (Middaugh et al. 1981).

A third finding from studies of animal behavior is that prenatal exposure to phenobarbital reduces the performance rates of mice being reinforced on a fixed ratio schedule (Middaugh, Santos, & Zemp 1975b). These results are not easy to interpret, but they seem to demonstrate that prenatal exposure to PB can have a detrimental effect on learned behavior later in the life of the animal.

Rats exposed to phenobarbital before birth are easily distracted by irrelevant stimuli during a shock escape task (Martin et al. 1979). On maze-learning tasks, PB-treated rats make more errors and take more time to learn the maze (Armitage 1952). However, the response decrement on maze tasks is not specific to offspring of females exposed to PB during pregnancy; nicotine, for instance, has similar effects (Peters & Ngan 1982). PB-exposed mice and rats also seem to be slower to learn avoidance responses (Formenti & Gamba 1980), but again, nicotine has similar effects. In short, there is little doubt that PB exposure during early development has a detrimental effect on learning, but the effects seem not to be unique to PB.

Additional study of the effects of prenatal exposure to phenobarbital on the acquisition of complex behavior is needed. Future research efforts should include cross-drug comparisons, improved behavioral tests, and cross-species comparisons of prenatal drug-exposure effects. Such research should answer many questions about pharmacological mechanisms of action in the fetus and clarify the causal relationship between fetal drug exposure and childhood learning disabilities.

REFERENCES

Armitage, S. G. 1952. The effects of barbiturates on the behavior of rat offspring as measured in learning and reasoning situations. *Journal of Comparative Physiology and Psychology* 45:146-152.

48 *Interdisciplinary Perspectives on Learning Disabilities*

Clemens, L. G., Popham, T. V., & Ruppert, P. H. 1979. Neonatal treatment of hamsters with barbiturate alters adult sexual behavior. *Developmental Psychobiology* 12:49-59.

Diaz, J., Schain, R. J., & Bailey, B. G. 1977. Phenobarbital-induced brain growth retardation in artificially reared rat pups. *Biology of the Neonate* 32:77-82.

Formenti, E. F., & Gamba, A. 1980. Behavioral tests in peri- and postnatal toxicity study in rats of trithiozine (Tresanil). *Archives of Toxicology* 4:284-287 (supplement).

Gupta, C., Shapiro, B. H., & Yaffe, S. In press. Prenatal exposure to phenobarbital: Decreased perinatal testosterone with subsequent reproductive dysfunction in male rats.

Gupta, C., Sonawane, B. R., & Yaffe, S. J. 1980. Phenobarbital exposure in utero: Alternations in female reproductive function in rats. *Science* 208:508-510.

Heinonen, O. P., Slone, D., & Shapiro, S. 1977. *Birth defects and drugs in pregnancy.* Littleton, MA: Publishing Sciences Group.

Manning, D. E., Stout, A. G., & Zemp, J. W. 1971. Effects of maternal phenobarbital administration on some aspects of neonatal brain development. *Federation Proceedings* 30:239.

Martin, J. C., Martin, D. C., Lamire, R., & Madder, B. 1979. Effects of maternal absorption of phenobarbital upon rat offspring development and function. *Neurobehavioral Toxicology* 1:49-55.

Middaugh, L. D., Blackwell, A. L., Boggan, W., & Zemp, J. W. 1981. Brain concentrations of phenobarbital and behavioral activation or depression. *Pharmacology, Biochemistry and Behavior* 15:723-728.

Middaugh, L. D., Drake, S. T., Fraley, J. E., & Zemp, J. W. 1972. Effects of subanesthetic doses of phenobarbital administered to pregnant mice on behavior of offspring. *Federation Proceedings* 31:595.

Middaugh, L. D., Santos, C. A., & Zemp, J. W. 1975a. Effects of phenobarbital given to pregnant mice on behavior of mature offspring. *Developmental Psychobiology* 8:305-313.

Middaugh, L. D., Santos, C. A., & Zemp, J. W. 1975b. Phenobarbital during pregnancy alters operant behavior of offspring in C57BL/6J mice. *Pharmacology, Biochemistry and Behavior* 3:1137-1139.

Middaugh, L. D., Simpson, L. W., Thomas, T. N., & Zemp, J. W. 1981. Prenatal maternal phenobarbital increases reactivity and retards habituation of mature offspring to environmental stimuli. *Psychopharmacology* 74:349-352.

Nichols, P. L., & Chen, T-C. 1981. *Minimal brain dysfunction: A prospective study.* Hillsdale, NJ: Erlbaum.

Peters, M. A., & Ngan, L. L. 1982. The effects of totigestational exposure to nicotine on pre- and postnatal development in the rat. *Archives Internationales Pharmacodynamie et de Therapie* 257(1):155-167.

Reinisch, J. M., & Sanders, S. A. 1982. Early barbiturate exposure: The brain, sexually dimorphic behavior and learning. *Neuroscience and Biobehavioral Reviews* 6:311-319.

Yanai, J., & Bergman, A. 1981. Neuronal deficits after neonatal exposure to phenobarbital. *Exploratory Neurology* 73:199-208.

Zemp, J. W., & Middaugh, L. D. 1975. Some effects of prenatal exposure to D-amphetamine sulfate and phenobarbital on developmental neurochemistry and on behavior. *Addiction Disorders* 2:307-331.

SMOKING AND DRINKING

Ann Pytkowicz Streissguth, Ph.D.

Research on the childhood effects of nicotine and alcohol use during pregnancy presents the same problems as research on the effects of prescription and nonprescription drugs. Smoking and drinking are common habits; in addition, many women who smoke also drink, and vice versa. Other methodological difficulties also make the existing epidemiological findings hard to interpret.

Chronic maternal alcoholism produces fetal alcohol syndrome, a common cause of mental retardation, in about one-third of exposed babies. Recent research suggests that moderate alcohol use may also be damaging, but learning disabilities per se have not been systematically studied. Dr. Streissguth's ongoing Pregnancy and Health Study, which provides for evaluation of the children of smokers and drinkers periodically to at least school age, should add much to our understanding of prenatal exposure to alcohol and nicotine.

Although we used to assume that the placenta protected the embryo and fetus from toxic substances, it is now clear that the placenta could be better represented as a sieve than a wall. Most common drugs cross the placenta readily (including both alcohol and nicotine) and circulation levels in fetal blood are often similar to those in maternal blood. Therefore, all ingestants of the mother, including diet, are important variables in determining the intrauterine environment. Not only are drugs important individually as possible teratogens, but one must also consider the possibility of drug interactions.

In studies with laboratory animals, nicotine and alcohol independently have been related to behavioral effects and performance, including delayed development, hyperactivity, and learning decrements. Behavioral effects have been observed at levels of exposure lower than those producing structural anomalies. Research on laboratory animals helps to establish a causal link between prenatal exposure and offspring effects. Findings from human studies, though more pertinent to childhood learning disorders, are more clouded with methodological problems.

Is prenatal exposure to alcohol or nicotine related to learning disabilities in school-age children? If we assume the usual definition of learning disabilities as performance in reading, spelling, or arithmetic at two or more grades below expectation, given normal intellectual capacity and adequate opportunity to learn, then no studies that I have been able to find address this question directly. However, many studies have investigated the long-term association between maternal smoking and drinking during pregnancy and various aspects of child behavior and development that may relate to learning disabilities, and these will now be reviewed.

Smoking

Cigarette smoking during pregnancy is known to be associated with low birthweight, prematurity, spontaneous abortion, stillbirth, and congenital anomalies (Pirani 1978, Abel 1980, Fried & Ohorn 1980, Johnston 1981, Martin 1982). Other effects of smoking on infant behavior include decreased fetal breathing movements and low Apgar scores, poor auditory habituation and orientation, and lower mental and motor test scores in infancy (Sontag & Wallace 1935, Garn et al. 1980, 1981, Saxton 1978).

Data relating behavior during childhood to maternal smoking come chiefly from three large-scale longitudinal studies. The first is the British Child Development Study, which collected data on 16,994 children born during the week of the Queen's birthday in 1958. The second is the Collaborative Perinatal Project, conducted between 1959 and 1974 on some 53,000 mother-child pairs in the United States. The third is the Canadian Prospective Study, an ongoing project comparing 168 low birthweight infants with 151 full birthweight controls.

Analyses of data from these and other studies show a relationship between cigarette smoking during pregnancy and the following childhood behavioral and performance measures: decrements in reading, arithmetic, general abilities, and IQ; learning difficulties; hyperactivity; impulsivity; neurological soft signs; and hyperkinesis (Butler & Goldstein 1973, Broman, Nichols, & Kennedy 1975, Nichols & Chen 1981, Dunn et al. 1976).

However, none of these studies adjusted for alcohol use, which is usually highly correlated with smoking, and most did not consider the important variables, such as social class, maternal education, and birth order, which have been shown to relate to these same outcomes. One might conclude that the weight of the evidence at this point favors some long-term sequelae, but whether they are related to smoking, alcohol, or both awaits further study.

Fetal Alcohol Syndrome

Unlike smoking, intrauterine alcohol exposure produces a recognizable pattern of malformation in the children who are most severely affected. Fetal alcohol syndrome (FAS) is a pattern of growth deficiency, dysmorphic facial characteristics, central nervous system dysfunction, and often a major malformation such as a heart defect. Children diagnosed as showing fetal alcohol syndrome are usually growth deficient at birth and continue to be so during childhood, which often makes them look younger than they are.

The most debilitating characteristic of FAS is mental retardation. A diagnosis of FAS in early infancy seems to carry a high risk of borderline to retarded mental development (Darby, Streissguth, & Smith 1981) although the range of intellectual function in individual cases is great. Figure 7 shows a severely retarded FAS child in early infancy, late infancy, and childhood.

The risk of having a child with FAS appears to be about one-third among chronic alcoholic mothers who drink during pregnancy, but so far the factors determining which children will be affected have not been identified. The frequency of FAS has been estimated at about one in 750 to 1,000 births, based on studies in Seattle, France, and Sweden. This makes FAS the third largest known cause of mental retardation. (Dehaene et al. 1981, Olegard et al. 1979, Hanson, Streissguth, & Smith 1978).

Fetal alcohol syndrome represents only one end of a continuum of alcohol-related birth defects. Several studies suggest that there are a spectrum of effects (Olegard et al. 1979, Hanson, Streissguth, & Smith 1978, Smith 1980, Majewski 1981), although in the absence of the full syndrome their identification in individual cases is often difficult.

Children of Alcoholic Mothers

If we consider FAS as one end of a continuum of fetal alcohol effects, the question of the IQ and development of children of alcoholic mothers in general needs to be addressed. Unfortunately, not many relevant studies have been done. Those that have suggest that maternal alcoholism does have a

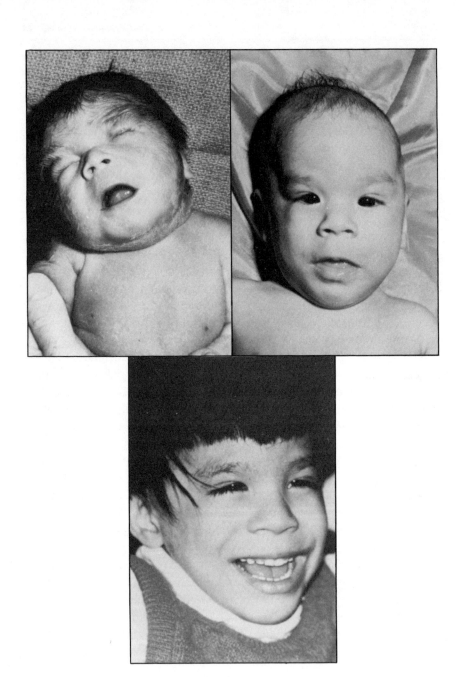

Figure 7. The child of a chronically alcoholic mother, diagnosed at birth as showing fetal alcohol syndrome. Although raised his entire life in one excellent foster home and a participant in various stimulation and remediation programs, he continues to have an IQ around 45 (more severe retardation than most FAS children) with accompanying hyperactivity and distractibility.

detrimental effect on children's IQ scores (Jones et al. 1974, Streissguth et al. 1979).

The importance of a history of alcohol abuse as a possible contributing factor in learning disabilities has been pointed out by a recent study (Shaywitz, Cohen, & Shaywitz 1980). Of 87 children referred to the Yale Learning Disorders Unit during a ten-month period, fifteen were born to mothers who were alcoholic during the pregnancy. Despite intellectual functioning in the normal to dull-normal range (the mean IQ was 98), all these children had been referred for school failure and all but one were hyperactive. Each child displayed at least two of the characteristic features of FAS. Almost half the children of these alcoholic mothers were below the fifth percentile for height, and one-fifth were below the third percentile for head circumference. This study contributes to our understanding of the broad range of possible alcohol-related disabilities in children and suggests the need to look beyond mental retardation and growth deficiency when examining outcomes.

The Pregnancy and Health Study

Since 1974, a longitudinal prospective study of 500 children preselected from a sample of 1,500 pregnant women to maximize the number of heavier drinkers and smokers has been carried out in Seattle (Streissguth et al. 1981). The goal of the study is to evaluate the long-term behavioral effects on offspring of maternal alcohol and cigarette use during pregnancy.

In a recent paper (Streissguth, Barr, & Martin 1982), we reported that at birth, Apgar scores were significantly lower for offspring of heavier drinkers but not for heavier smokers. Alcohol use was also significantly related to heart-rate abnormalities in the newborn, and to respiratory distress. At one and two days of age, using the Brazelton Neonatal Assessment Scale, significant alcohol effects on habituation and arousal were found, even when statistical adjustments were made for nicotine, caffeine, birth order, sex, and age of infants. At eight months, we found small but statistically significant alcohol-related decrements on both the mental and motor Bayley Infant Scales (Streissguth et al. 1980). Nicotine was not significantly related to these outcomes.

When the children had reached four years of age, alcohol and nicotine independently were found to be associated with poor performance on a laboratory vigilance task measuring attention. While we cannot yet say what the long-range implications of these early deficits might be, we hope that systematic follow-up of these children as they grow will clarify the contribution of intrauterine alcohol and nicotine exposure to childhood learning disabilities.

Another follow-up study of four-year-old children born to mothers interviewed during pregnancy identified small but statistically significant alcohol-related decrements in focused attention through naturalistic observations in the child's home (Landesman-Dwyer, Ragozin, & Little 1981). This study is noteworthy in that only mothers reporting a moderate level of alcohol intake (about one drink a day on the average) were included; all heavy drinkers were deleted from the sample. The findings point up the need for continued investigation of the effects of moderate as well as heavy alcohol used during pregnancy.

The many types and subtypes of learning disabilities could well be our most sensitive indicators of the long-term consequences of intrauterine exposure to toxic substances. However, the long-term studies necessary to delineate these relationships are time-consuming, tedious, and expensive. Furthermore, a host of methodologic problems can operate against the demonstration of positive results. So little is known about the etiology of childhood learning disabilities that we cannot even be sure of the proper models to follow. In our Pregnancy and Health Study, for example, we hypothesized a relationship between learning disabilities and alcohol exposure because clear mental retardation can exist in the most severely affected cases. Is it logical to expect that lower doses or different patterns of alcohol use will be related to smaller functional decrements?

The answers to these and related questions are as yet unknown. Although finding them will be difficult, research on the prevention of learning disabilities is of the utmost importance. Clearly the time is ripe for the collaboration of basic scientists and educators for the improved welfare of children.

REFERENCES

Abel, E. L. 1980. Smoking during pregnancy: A review of effects on growth and development of offspring. *Human Biology* 52:593-625.

Broman, S. H., Nichols, P. L., & Kennedy, W. A. 1975. *Preschool IQ: Prenatal and early developmental correlates.* Hillsdale, NJ, Erlbaum.

Butler, N. R., & Goldstein, H. 1973. Smoking in pregnancy and subsequent child development. *British Medical Journal* 4:573-575.

Darby, B. L., Streissguth, A. P., & Smith, D. W. 1981. A preliminary follow-up of 8 children diagnosed fetal alcohol syndrome in infancy. *Neurobehavioral Toxicology and Teratology* 3:157-159.

Dehaene, P., Crepin, G., Delahousse, G., Querleu, D., Walbaum, R., Titran, M., & Samaille-Villette, C. 1981. Aspects epidemiologiques du syndrome d'alcoolisme foetal. *La Nouvelle Presse Medicale* 10:2639-2643.

Dunn, H. G., McBurney, A. K., Ingram, S., & Hunter, C. M. 1976.

Maternal cigarette smoking during pregnancy and the child's subsequent development: I. Physical growth to the age of 6½ years. *Canadian Journal of Public Health* 67:499-505.

Fried, P., & Ohorn, H. 1980. *Smoking for two: Cigarettes and pregnancy.* New York: Free Press.

Garn, S. M., Petzold, A. S., Ridella, S. A., & Johnston, M. 1980. Effect of smoking during pregnancy on Apgar and Bayley scores. *Lancet* 2:912-913.

Garn, S. M., Johnston, M., Ridella, S. A., & Petzold, A. S. 1981. Effect of maternal cigarette smoking on Apgar scores. *American Journal of Diseases of Children* 135:503-506.

Hanson, J. W., Streissguth, A. P., & Smith, D. W. 1978. Effects of moderate alcohol consumption during pregnancy on fetal growth and morphogenesis. *Journal of Pediatrics* 92:457-460.

Johnston, C. 1981. Cigarette smoking and the outcome of human pregnancies: A status report on the consequences. *Clinical Toxicology* 18:189-209.

Jones, K. L., Smith, D. W., Streissguth, A. P., & Myrianthopoulos, N. C. 1974. Outcome in offspring of chronic alcoholic women. *Lancet* 1:1076-1078.

Landesman-Dwyer, S., Ragozin, A. S., & Little, R. E. 1981. Behavioral correlates of prenatal alcohol exposure: A four-year follow-up study. *Neurobehavioral Toxicology and Teratology* 3:187-193.

Majewski, F. 1981. Alcohol embryopathy: Some facts and speculations about pathogenesis. *Neurobehavioral Toxicology and Teratology* 3:129-144.

Martin, J. C. 1982. An overview: Maternal nicotine and caffeine consumption and offspring outcome. *Neurobehavioral Toxicology and Teratology* 4:421-427.

Nichols, P. L., & Chen, T-C. 1981. *Minimal brain dysfunction: A prospective study.* Hillsdale, NJ: Erlbaum.

Olegard, R., Sabel, K. G., Aronsson, M., Sandin, B., Johansson, P. R., Carlsson, C., Kyllerman, M., Iversen, K., & Hrbek, A. 1979. Effects on the child of alcohol abuse during pregnancy. *Acta Paedicatrica Scandinavica Supplement* (Stockholm) 275:112-121.

Pirani, B. B. K. 1978. Smoking during pregnancy. *Obstetrical & Gynecological Survey* 33:1-13.

Saxton, D. W. 1978. The behavior of infants whose mothers smoke in pregnancy. *Early Human Development* 2:363-369.

Shaywitz, S. E., Cohen, D. J., & Shaywitz, B. A. 1980. Behavior and learning difficulties in children of normal intelligence born to alcoholic mothers. *Journal of Pediatrics* 96:978-982.

Smith, D. W. 1980. Alcohol effects on the fetus. In R. H. Schwartz & S. J. Yaffe (Eds.), *Drug and chemical risks to the fetus and newborn.* New York: Alan R. Liss.

Sontag, L. W., & Wallace, R. F. 1935. The effect of cigarette smoking during pregnancy upon the fetal heart rate. *American Journal of Obstetrics and Gynecology* 29:77-83.

Streissguth, A. P., Barr, H. M., & Martin, D. C. 1982. Offspring effects and pregnancy complications related to self-reported maternal use. *Developmental Pharmacology and Therapeutics* 5:21-32.

Streissguth, A. P., Barr, H. M., Martin, D. C., & Herman, C. S. 1980. Effects of maternal alcohol, nicotine, and caffeine use during pregnancy on infant development at 8 months. *Alcoholism: Clinical and Experimental Research* 4:152-164.

Streissguth, A. P., Little, R. E., Herman, C., & Woodell, S. 1979. IQ of children of recovered alcoholic mothers compared to matched controls. *Alcoholism: Clinical and Experimental Research* 3:197.

Streissguth, A. P., Martin, D. C., Martin, J. C., & Barr, H. M. 1981. The Seattle longitudinal prospective study on alcohol and pregnancy. *Neurobehavioral Toxicology and Teratology* 3:223-233.

OBSTETRIC MEDICATIONS

Sarah H. Broman, Ph.D.

Most obstetric medications quickly enter the circulatory system of the fetus via the placenta. The effects of these medications on newborns have been studied extensively, and many—including Demerol, and local and inhalation anesthetics—have been found to depress neonatal physiological and behavioral responses. Data on the long-term effects of obstetric drugs is much less plentiful, and differences and methodological problems in research design complicate the comparison and interpretation of findings from different studies.

Dr. Broman describes nine studies assessing the effects of obstetric medications on children past infancy, including three that focused on learning disabilities specifically. Several of these studies suggest that inhalation anesthetics at delivery place children at risk for cognitive deficits, including learning disabilities. Labor induction by oxytocin and the use of scopolamine may also have long-term effects. However, further follow-up studies on children are needed to confirm these findings and to assess other relationships between intrapartum drugs and later cognitive development. In the meantime, the American Academy of Pediatrics recommends that obstetricians avoid some drugs and administer the lowest effective doses of others for pain relief during labor and delivery.

Ideally, this review should address three questions. First, do the effects of drugs used in labor and delivery persist beyond the perinatal period? Second, are these effects evident in the performance of cognitive, perceptual, or attentional tasks? Third, if there is evidence for the second point, can the children showing cognitive dysfunctions be characterized as learning disabled, that is, as having normal aptitude or IQ scores and unexpectedly poor academic performance? Not surprisingly, these questions cannot now be answered satisfactorily.

Most behavioral studies of the effects of drugs used in childbirth are concentrated in the newborn period. Only a handful provide information on children over one year of age, and of these only three address learning disabilities specifically, rather than more general patterns of cognitive or behavioral development. After a brief review of neonatal drug effects, these studies of older children will be described.

Drug Effects on Neonates

With few exceptions, drugs used in obstetric anesthesia and analgesia rapidly cross the placenta and enter the fetal circulation (Perriss 1981, Shnider 1981). The ability of the neonate to metabolize many drugs is poorly developed, so that the effects of drugs given during labor may persist after delivery, when elimination through the maternal circulation is no longer possible (Beeley 1981).

Table 5 lists the types of drugs commonly used during labor and delivery. Narcotics, barbiturates and other sedatives, and inhalation anesthetics are all known to cause respiratory depression in the newborn, at least briefly (e.g., Morselli & Rovei 1980, James 1975). Other negative outcomes associated with these drugs include alterations in heart rate, lowered Apgar scores, and abnormal patterns of sleep and wakefulness. Local anesthetics can cause minimal depression in the newborn but increase the frequency of operative deliveries by reducing the mother's ability to bear down. The local anesthetic lidocaine is also associated with abnormal fetal heart rate patterns. Unless used carefully, drugs that induce or augment labor can produce contractions that are too strong and sustained for the safety of mother and child;

as will be indicated below, oxytocin appears to carry more risk than the prostaglandins.

Table 5. Common Obstetric Medications

Narcotics	Inhalation anesthetics
Alphaprodine (Nisentil)	Halothane
Meperidine (Demerol)	Nitrous oxide
	Local anesthetics (spinal,
Barbiturates	caudal, and epidural blocks)
Secobarbital	Bupivacaine
Thiopental	Lidocaine
Other sedative—hypnotics	Inductive drugs
Diazepam (Valium)	Oxytocin
Scopolamine	Prostaglandins

Most studies of behavioral (as contrasted with physiological) drug effects on newborns have also identified depression of function. For example, a study on the effects of meperidine using the Brazelton Neonatal Assessment Scale (Belsey et al. 1981) found that this drug was associated with depressed attention and social responsiveness throughout the first six weeks of life, although the changes observed were relatively subtle. In another study using the Brazelton scale (Aleksandrowicz & Aleksandrowicz 1974), the infant behaviors most affected by pain-relieving drugs (anesthetics and analgesics) were habituation, orientation, cuddliness, and smiles, and the drugs showing the strongest relationships to outcome were tranquilizers, barbiturates, and a neuromuscular blocking agent. Some of these relationships were most marked at one month of age (when the study ended), implying persistent impairment of function.

Obstetric medications have been shown to affect not only test performance but various discrete behavioral responses in newborns. Depressed sucking and feeding in the first days of life have been associated with anesthetics (Dubignon et al. 1969) and barbiturates (Brazelton 1961, Kron, Stein, & Goddard 1966).

Cognitive-Behavioral Outcomes in Children

Of nine studies relating obstetric medication to outcome past one year of age, only three used children classified as having learning disorders as subjects. The other six studies investigated cognitive development in children unselected for learning problems. Within the latter group, three studies yielded positive findings (that is, identified drug-associated deficits in cognitive functioning). The other three showed no childhood drug effects.

In the first of the three general studies with positive results, Muller and colleagues (1971) investigated the relationship of perinatal factors to mental development and school achievement at age nine in a sample of 1,700 children born in 1956. The primary finding was a relationship between breech delivery and poor school performance. In addition, lower birthweight and inhalation anesthesia at delivery were both related to slightly but significantly lower scores on the Lorge-Thorndike intelligence test.

A second study found an association between oxytocin-induced labor and otherwise unexplained language and motor delays at about four years of age (Friedman, Sachtleben, & Wallace 1979). Prostaglandin induction did not seem to have adverse effects.

Third, a prospectively designed study from the Collaborative Perinatal Project has examined relationships between obstetric medication and physical and cognitive development through age seven (Broman 1981, Broman & Brackbill 1980). The subjects were 1,944 full-term infants of normal birthweight, born to mothers with uncomplicated pregnancies and vaginal vertex deliveries. The pharmacological agents evaluated were inhalation anesthetics and six other drugs. Outcomes were assessed in the first year of life through pediatric examinations at birth and at four months, a psychomotor test with the Bayley Scales at eight months, and a pediatric neurological examination at one year. At ages four and seven, psychometric examinations that included an intelligence test were administered.

Considering behavioral outcomes only, the results suggest that in the first year of life inhalation anesthetics and oxytocin are both related to psychomotor deficits. Inhalants are also associated with poor neuromotor functioning. At older ages, the most consistent findings involved scopolamine, oxytocin, and inhalation anesthetics. Scopolamine was negatively associated with performance on some intelligence test items at four and seven years. Oxytocin was associated with lower fine motor scores at age four and with lower reading, spelling, and verbal analogies scores at age seven. Inhalants were associated with behavior that could be characterized as socially withdrawn.

These findings suggest hypotheses that require independent confirmation. Because a large number of covariates were included in each analysis, overcontrolling rather than confounding may be the major analytic problem. However, some of the significant associations found could be due to chance. A drug-free control group of sufficient size was not available for comparative study—a common difficulty confronting investigators of drug effects.

The studies of general cognitive development producing negative results efly summarized. First, DeCoster and colleagues (1981) replicated ng cited earlier concerning the absence of deleterious effects follow- or induced by prostaglandins. Second, Ounsted and colleagues (1980) perinatal factors to be unrelated to motor abilities, language, or comprehension at age four in a sample of 570 children. Third, a prospective investigation of the long-term effects of obstetric medication in approximately 4,000 children from the Oakland area found no significant effect of anesthesia or analgesia on cognitive development at age five (Dailey et al. 1982). A separate report on this study reported no differences among groups of five-year-olds whose mothers had received different analgesic drugs or between these groups and controls (van den Berg 1981).

Children with Learning Disabilities

In the three studies investigating relationships between obstetric medication and learning handicaps specifically, there is considerable variation in methodology and in sophistication of approach. In a retrospective study (Colletti 1979), events in the birth records of 50 learning disabled children between the ages of seven and twelve were compared with those reported in a descriptive study of 39,000 mothers and infants enrolled in the Collaborative Perinatal Project (Niswander & Gordon 1972). A higher frequency of pregnancy and birth complications was found in the sample of children that had been referred for learning problems than in the "normative population." The variable relevant to this review was induction of labor (method unspecified), which had a frequency of 24 percent in the study sample compared with an estimated normal rate of 10 percent.

In another retrospective study, the obstetric histories of 70 kibbutz children diagnosed as having minimal brain dysfunction (MBD) at age nine were compared with those of a control group matched for age and sex (Kaffman, Sivan-Sher, & Carel 1981). Medications in labor and delivery were more frequent in the MBD than in the control group, as were complications of pregnancy and delivery, low and high birthweights, and shorter gestational age. Also more frequent in the MBD group were chronic maternal illness, drugs prescribed during pregnancy, and newborn complications. The major difference between groups in obstetric medication was a fourfold increase in inhalation anesthetics in the MBD group.

The third investigation of learning disabled children is a prospective one from the Collaborative Perinatal Project. The development of 994 low achievers was followed from the prenatal period through age seven (Broman, Bien, & Shaughnessy in press). These children met the study criteria of normal aptitude or intelligence test scores at age seven and below-average academic achievement. Full-scale IQ on the Wechsler Intelligence Scale for

Children was at least 90, and reading or spelling score on the Wide Range Achievement Test was more than one year below grade placement. Low achievers were compared with IQ-matched academically successful controls of the same ethnic group on medical-biological, psychological, and social characteristics.

Inhalation anesthetics at delivery was a significant perinatal discriminator between low achievers and controls in the white sample. Frequencies in the two groups were 42 percent and 29 percent, respectively. Inhalants remained significant in summary analyses of all early discriminators through age four and all discriminators through age seven. Controlling for hospital of birth failed to affect these results. Identical findings were obtained in a subgroup of more academically impaired low achievers; for this group, the frequency of inhalation anesthetics was 45 percent compared with 29 percent in controls. In the black sample, inhalation anesthetics were associated with hyperactivity among low achievers.

Considering the small number of long-term follow-up studies on obstetric drug effects, it is difficult to determine why some have positive and others negative findings (although there are obvious differences in study design). The positive findings in the three studies of learning disabilities, with two reporting a relationship with inhalants at delivery, are consistent with the view that learning handicaps are symptoms of neurological dysfunction resulting from complications in the perinatal period. But as Rourke (1978) has pointed out, while prenatal and perinatal complications are found more frequently in histories of children with learning disabilities, they provide neither a necessary nor a sufficient explanation.

Further Research

The high ratio of neonatal studies to follow-up studies in childhood demonstrates an immediate and striking need for further research on the long-term effects of obstetric analgesics and anesthetics. Drug-related deficits in neonatal responsiveness to the environment suggest the possibility of deficits in responsiveness or learning at later ages. As with the sequelae of other perinatal stresses, the physiological and behavioral depression of the drug-exposed neonate, even if not itself a critical sign, may be a precursor of developmental jeopardy at a later age (Lipsitt 1979).

From the pharmacological side, concern about possible long-term consequences of drugs given in labor and delivery stems from lack of knowledge about the effects of a given agent on the fetus or newborn even though the effects may be known in the adult. This issue has been emphasized in earlier reviews of obstetric medication and infant outcome. As has been pointed out in other papers, the immaturity of the central nervous system increases its vulnerability to insult. One consequence (suggested by Rodier 1980) that could have a variety of behavioral outcomes is interference with neuro-genesis in regions of the brain where neurons continue to proliferate after birth. Another mechanism that may underlie long-term effects of maternal analgesia and anesthesia is perinatal anoxia, a condition associated with lower cognitive functioning at later ages (Broman 1979, Gottfried 1973).

Concerns about known and unknown effects of drugs given in labor and delivery on the fetus and newborn have been formalized in a statement from the American Academy of Pediatrics (1978), which includes a call for further studies. Two committees of pediatricians and obstetricians jointly recommend avoidance of drugs or drug dosages known to produce significant changes in infant neurobehavior and the use of the minimum effective dose of analgesic or anesthetic agents when indicated for reasonable relief of pain.

REFERENCES

Aleksandrowicz, M. K., & Aleksandrowicz, D. R. 1974. Obstetrical pain-relieving drugs as predictors of infant behavior variability. *Child Development* 45:935-945.

American Academy of Pediatrics Committee on Drugs. 1978. Effect of medication during labor and delivery on infant outcome. *Pediatrics* 62:402-403.

Beeley, L. 1981. Adverse effects of drugs in later pregnancy. *Clinics in Obstetrics and Gynaecology* 8:275-290.

Belsey, E. M., Rosenblatt, D. B., Lieberman, B. A., Redshaw, M., Caldwell, J., Notarianni, L., Smith, R. L., & Beard, R. W. 1981. The influence of maternal analgesia on neonatal behaviour: I. Pethidine. *British Journal of Obstetrics and Gynaecology* 88:398-406.

Brazelton, T. B. 1961. Psychophysiologic reactions in the neonate. II. Effect of maternal medication on the neonate and his behavior. *Journal of Pediatrics* 58:513-518.

Broman, S. H. 1979. Perinatal anoxia and cognitive development in early childhood. In T. M. Field, A. M. Sostek, S. Goldberg, & H. H. Schuman (Eds.), *Infants born at risk: Behavior and development*. Jamaica, NY: Spectrum.

Broman, S. H. 1981. Risk factors for deficits in early cognitive development. In G. G. Berg & H. D. Maillie (Eds.), *Measurement of risks*. New York: Plenum.

Broman, S. H., Bien, E. C., & Shaughnessy, P. W. In press. *Unexpected school failure*. Hillsdale, NJ: Erlbaum.

Broman, S. H., & Brackbill, Y. 1980. Obstetric medication and early development. *Abstracts of Papers of the 146th National Meeting of the American Association for the Advancement of Science.* AAAS Publication 80-2:61.

Colletti, L. F. 1979. Relationship between pregnancy and birth complications and the later development of learning disabilities. *Journal of Learning Disabilities* 12:659-663.

Dailey, P. A., Baysinger, C. L., Levinson, G., & Shnider, S. M. 1982. Neurobehavioral testing of the newborn infant. *Clinics in Perinatology* 9:191-214.

DeCoster, W., Goethals, A., Vandierendonck, A., Thiery, M., & Derom, R. 1981. Effects of labour induction with prostaglandin F on the psychomotor development of the child in the first 30 months: A follow-up study of risk cases (Belgium). In S. A. Mednick & A. E. Baert (Eds.), *Perspective longitudinal research: An empirical basis for the primary prevention of psychosocial disorders.* New York: Oxford University Press.

Dubignon, J., Campbell, D., Curtis, M., & Partington, M. W. 1969. The relation between laboratory measures of sucking, food intake, and perinatal factors during the newborn period. *Child Development* 40:1107-1120.

Friedman, E. A., Sachtleben, M. R., & Wallace, A. K. 1979. Infant outcome following labor induction. *American Journal of Obstetrics and Gynecology* 133:718-722.

Gottfried, A. W. 1973. Intellectual consequences of perinatal anoxia. *Psychological Bulletin* 80:231-242.

James, F. M. 1975. Inhalation anesthetics. *Contemporary Obstetrics and Gynecology* 5:73-76.

Kaffman, M., Sivan-Sher, A., & Carel, C. 1981. Obstetric history of kibbutz children with minimal brain dysfunction. *Israeli Journal of Psychiatry and Related Sciences* 18:69-84.

Kron, R. E., Stein, M., & Goddard, K. E. 1966. Newborn sucking behavior affected by obstetric sedation. *Pediatrics* 37:1012-1016.

Lipsitt, L. P. 1979. Learning assessments and interventions for the infant born at risk. In T. M. Field, A. M. Sostek, S. Goldberg, & H. H. Schuman (Eds.), *Infants born at risk: Behavior and development.* Jamaica, NY: Spectrum.

Morselli, P. L., & Rovei, V. 1980. Placental transfer of pethidine and nor-pethidine and their pharmacokinetics in the newborn. *European Journal of Clinical Pharmacology* 18:25-30.

Muller, P. F., Campbell, H. E., Graham, W. E., Brittain, H., Fitzgerald, J. A., Hogan, M. A., Muller, V. H., & Rittenhouse, A. H. 1971. Perinatal factors and their relationship to mental retardation and other parameters of development. *American Journal of Obstetrics and Gynecology* 109:1205-1210.

Niswander, K. R., & Gordon, M. (Eds.). 1972. *The women and their pregnancies.* Philadelphia: Saunders.

Ounsted, M., Scott, A., & Moar, V. 1980. Delivery and development: To what extent can one associate cause and effect? *Journal of the Royal Society of Medicine* 73:786-792.

Perriss, B. W. 1981. Analgesia and anesthesia. *Clinics in Obstetrics and Gynaecology* 8:475-506.

Rodier, P. M. 1980. Chronology of neuron development: Animal studies and their clinical implications. *Developmental Medicine and Child Neurology* 22:525-545.

Rourke, B. P. 1978. Neuropsychological research in reading retardation: A review. In A. L. Benton & D. Pearl (Eds.), *Dyslexia—An appraisal of current knowledge.* New York: Oxford University Press.

Shnider, S. M. 1981. Choice of anesthesia for labor and delivery. *Obstetrics and Gynecology* 58:24S-34S (supplement).

van den Berg, B. J. 1981. Evaluation of long-term effects of obstetric medication. Paper presented at the Western Society for Pediatric Research, Carmel, CA.

OBSTETRICAL TRAUMA

Don C. Creevy, M.D.

The effects of obstetrical trauma, like those of obstetric medications, have been much more thoroughly studied in newborns than in older children. Even with newborns, however, outcome assessment is difficult, because several traumatic events often occur during the same delivery. Thus, although research indicates that complications of pregnancy and birth do put infants at risk for central nervous system damage, it does not provide good data on the amount of risk associated with individual hazards.

In general, Dr. Creevy says, research on long-term sequelae of obstetrical trauma does not prove or even strongly suggest that trauma causes learning disabilities, though neither does it rule out the possibility. In addition, studies of fetal asphyxia, which seems the most likely mechanism by which trauma might damage the brain, fail to support the concept of a continuum of reproductive casualty. Some infants who experience asphyxia at birth are seriously damaged; the great majority of the rest show no ill effects at all.

Nonetheless, Dr. Creevy believes that future studies may show a relationship between learning disabilities and various events at the time of labor and delivery. A practicing obstetrician and an avowed noninterventionist, he suggests that physicians avoid all unnecessary interference with the natural birth process and do everything possible to minimize trauma during complicated deliveries.

Subtle neurologic abnormalities are of uncertain origin, and there is little agreement about their definition. Terms such as learning disability, minimal brain dysfunction, attention deficit disorder, hyperactivity, dyslexia, and many others have been used to identify children of normal intelligence who are behaviorally different from their peers and who may have a history of prematurity or other pregnancy and birth complications.

Obstetrical trauma is equally difficult to define, and its *effects* are just as debatable as are the *causes* of learning disabilities. Obstetrical trauma is defined here as any event at the time of labor and delivery that could result in physical damage to the fetal nervous system, asphyxia of the fetus with resulting anoxia (strictly speaking, hypoxia) of the nervous system, or intoxication of the fetus with toxins or drugs taken by the mother.

Obstetric medications are discussed in the preceding paper and, though a common cause of trauma, will not be considered in detail here. A number of other important perinatal events are within the scope of this discussion but not found in the literature on learning disabilities. They include electronic fetal monitoring, artificial rupture of fetal membranes, immobilization of the laboring woman, nutritional deprivation in labor to prevent possible anesthetic complications, maternal hypotension or hyperventilation during labor, intrapartum infection due to prolonged rupture of membranes, frequent vaginal examinations in labor, and episiotomy.

Multiple Traumas

Often, several traumatic events occur during the same labor and delivery. An example is a difficult, emergency forceps delivery in a case of premature placental separation with fetal distress. The premature fetus is asphyxiated by loss of placental oxygen, intoxicated by an anesthetic agent, traumatized physically by the forceps and the maternal pelvis, and further asphyxiated by vasospasm and prolonged pressure on and swelling of the brain. The effects of these many events are extremely difficult to separate for study.

An Israeli kibbutz study compared 70 children with diagnosed minimal brain dysfunction (MBD) with 70 age- and sex-matched control subjects (Kaffman, Sivan-Sher, & Carel 1981). The mean age was 9½ years, with a ratio of 2.8 boys to 1 girl. Socioeconomic status for the group was very uniform. The investigators found statistically significant differences between the two groups in complications of pregnancy; complications of labor and delivery; medications used in pregnancy, labor, and delivery; birthweight; and gestational age. Complications of labor and delivery, including prolonged labor with fetal distress, use of forceps and vacuum extraction, and cesarean section, were associated almost exclusively with the MBD group.

The authors concluded that pregnancy and birth complications put infants at risk for central nervous system damage. However, they further stated:

> We found that, for the great majority of MBD children in our sample who have a positive history of pregnancy and/or birth complications, no one single, risk-evolving factor is involved, but a combination of several potential pathogenic influences and hazards during the intrauterine and newborn periods. The interaction of two or more noxious factors working together at a point in time, and also in combination throughout various developmental stages of the fetus, greatly hampers any attempt to evaluate the relative roles of the isolated factors.

The classic work of Kawi and Pasamanick (1958), the first major study of the relationship between perinatal factors and childhood reading disorders, found more premature births and more complications of pregnancy and birth (especially maternal preeclampsia, hypertensive disease, and placental abnormalities) among poor readers than in control groups. However, a critical research review by Balow and colleagues (1975-76) states that "the literature cited by Kawi and Pasamanick, contrary to their interpretation, offers little or no support for the hypothesis that reading failure is especially related to anomalous events of pregnancy and birth."

Some Specific Obstetrical Traumas

Many articles have been published concerning the effects on the newborn infant of asphyxia, dysfunctional labor, abnormal presentations, obstetrical forceps, and the vacuum extractor. Long-term follow-up studies are rare, and in general they do not assess learning disabilities as a possible outcome of a specific form of trauma.

After a brief review of fetal asphyxia, Niswander (1979) concluded, "While fetal asphyxia clearly *can* cause fetal brain damage, the infrequency of this relationship is stressed." Niswander and colleagues (1975) studied children from the Collaborative Perinatal Project who had been subject to hypoxia in association with premature placental separation, placenta praevia, and compression of the umbilical cord. They compared their IQ and motor function at four years to that of matched controls and found no differences between the experimental and control groups.

In another investigation, Thompson and colleagues (1977) studied 31 children who suffered severe birth asphyxia over five to ten years. Seven percent were severely disabled and mentally retarded; the remainder had no serious handicap and were psychologically indistinguishable from the controls. The researchers were unable to identify any perinatal events that were predictive of an adverse outcome. They concluded, "The quality of life enjoyed by the large majority of the survivors was such as to justify a positive approach to the resuscitation of very severe asphyxiated neonates."

These and other recent studies suggest that intrapartum hypoxia causes a nearly all-or-nothing effect, resulting in either death or severe injury (cerebral palsy or severe retardation) on the one hand or no detectable injury on the other. They do *not* support the concept of a continuum of reproductive casualty as first postulated by Lilienfeld and Parkhurst (1951). However, neither do they impair its value as an epidemiological tool (Nelson 1968). Perhaps we still lack sufficiently sensitive measuring techniques, and as they are developed the concept will be found to be valid.

Breech delivery, especially when carried out vaginally, has long been known to be associated with increased perinatal morbidity and mortality. In recent years, the use of cesarean for breech delivery has been widely advocated even though maternal mortality is increased from two to thirty times by cesarean section (Evrard & Gold 1977). Fianu and Joelsson (1979) found a much lower learning disabilities rate among breech infants born by cesarean than among those born vaginally, though the pattern of findings as a whole in this investigation is difficult to interpret.

Little has been written about the long-term, subtle effects on the child of the use of forceps and the vacuum extractor. Historically, the use of forceps has been associated with severe trauma to mother and baby. This is because, before cesarean section became relatively safe, it was the only possible means of effecting delivery in many difficult cases. Today, forceps are most commonly used to overcome the effects of regional anesthesia or to help an exhausted mother who needs the slightest added force to complete her delivery. Most obstetricians have discarded the difficult midforceps operation in favor of cesarean section (Paintin 1982).

Nelson and Broman (1977) studied 50 severely retarded children from the Collaborative Perinatal Project at age seven. Labor and delivery factors that distinguished between these children and normal controls were lowest fetal heart rate, arrested progress of labor, and use of midforceps. Intracranial hemorrhage at birth and neonatal seizures were the best predictors of severe, prolonged neurological handicap.

Establishing Causal Relationships

The studies reviewed remind us of the fragility of the fetal head and brain, especially in the premature infant, and underscore the importance of avoiding hypoxia and physical trauma at birth. They do not prove or even suggest strongly that learning disabilities are caused by hypoxia and trauma.

It does not appear that the ideal study of the relationship between perinatal factors and learning disabilities has been carried out. The long-term goals of such a study would be (1) prevention of the development of learning disabilities in as many children as possible, and (2) early identification of children at risk to permit remediation before more damage is done.

The ideal study would be prospective. It would guarantee absolute standardization of all medical records for mother and infant, very clear and circumscribed definitions of terms, and adequate control of variables other than those under study. The study would require a control group of infants born to *true* normals: healthy women who were able to go through pregnancy, labor, delivery, and lactation with an absolute minimum of artificial intervention based on medical or social custom. Babies whose mothers received drugs in pregnancy or labor, or who were delivered by forceps or cesarean, would *not* qualify as controls. These interventions themselves may have a negative impact on the child's brain integrity or may act synergistically with obstetrical traumas of natural or iatrogenic origin to confound the causal relationships.

Predicting the development of learning disabilities in a neonate or young child is probably even more difficult than establishing their relationship to obstetrical trauma. In most studies, relatively few of the infants who were subjected to an adverse perinatal event developed identifiable neurologic sequelae, even though the event may have increased the probability. Combinations of events seem to have greater predictive value than single events.

In addition, a good child-rearing environment may mask or even negate the effects of a traumatic birth. In a provocative review of the literature on the relationship between perinatal factors and the ultimate cognitive competence of children, Sameroff (1979) emphasized the importance of socioeconomic status and the quality of caretaking in overcoming the adverse effects of birth complications. He proposed "a continuum of caretaking casualty to incorporate the environmental risk factors leading toward poor developmental outcomes" and continued, "although reproductive casualties may play an initiating role in the production of later problems, it is the caretaking environment that determines the ultimate outcome."

Iatrogenesis

Despite the lack of evidence at present, it is conceivable that there is a causal relationship between certain perinatal events and learning disabilities. If so, it follows that a physician who causes such a perinatal event has increased the probability of occurrence of the learning disabilities. An obvious example is the case of an ill-planned induction of labor or elective repeat cesarean in which the baby turns out to be premature. The physician, by causing the infant to be born prematurely, has subjected the baby to an increased risk of all kinds of problems, including learning disabilities.

In my opinion, obstetrical interventions in general should be minimized or abandoned unless and until they have been demonstrated to be both beneficial and sufficiently safe that their benefits outweigh their risks. It does not appear that the future learning disabled child can yet be identified through neonatal neurobehavioral examination. Still, the obstetrician may be able to have some small impact on the future incidence of learning disabilities by acting in several ways: to decrease the incidence of prematurity; minimize the use of drugs in pregnancy, labor, and delivery; avoid or treat aggressively conditions that lead to hypoxia in utero; avoid traumatic delivery; and foster positive maternal attitudes toward pregnancy, birth, and the new child.

REFERENCES

Balow, B., Rubin, R., & Rosen, M. 1975-76. Perinatal events as precursors of reading disability. *Reading Research Quarterly* 11:36-71.

Evrard, J. R., & Gold, E. M. 1977. Cesarean section and maternal mortality in Rhode Island. *Obstetrics and Gynecology* 50:594-597.

Fianu, S., & Joelsson, I. 1979. Minimal brain dysfunction in children born in breech presentation. *Acta Obstetrica Gynecologica Scandinavica* 58:295-299.

Kaffman, M., Sivan-Sher, A., & Carel, C. 1981. Obstetrical history of kibbutz children with minimal brain dysfunction. *Israeli Journal of Psychiatry and Related Sciences* 18:69-84.

Kawi, A. A., & Pasamanick, B. 1958. Association of factors of pregnancy with learning disorders in childhood. *Journal of the American Medical Association* 166:1420-1423.

Lilienfeld, A. M., & Parkhurst, E. 1951. A study of the association of factors of pregnancy and parturition with the development of cerebral palsy: Preliminary report. *American Journal of Hygiene* 53:262-282.

Nelson, K. B. 1968. The "continuum of reproductive casualty." In R. MacKeith & M. Bax (Eds.), *Studies in infancy.* Oxford: Heinemann.

Nelson, K. B., & Broman, S. H. 1977. Perinatal risk factors in children with serious motor and mental handicaps. *Annals of Neurology* 2:371-377.

Niswander, K. R. 1979. The obstetrician, fetal asphyxia, and cerebral palsy. *American Journal of Obstetrics and Gynecology* 133:358-361.

Niswander, K. R., Gordon, M., & Drage, J. S. 1975. The effect of intrauterine hypoxia on the child surviving to 4 years. *American Journal of
Obstetrics & Gynecology* 121:892-899.

Paintin, D. B. 1982. Mid-cavity forceps delivery. *British Journal of
Obstetrics and Gynaecology* 89:495-500.

Sameroff, A. J. 1979. The etiology of cognitive competence: A systems
perspective. In R. B. Kearsley & I. E. Sigel (Eds.), *Infants at risk: Assessment of cognitive functioning.* Hillsdale, NJ: Erlbaum.

Thompson, A. J., Searle, M., & Russell, G. 1977. Quality of survival after
severe birth asphyxia. *Archives of Disease in Childhood* 52:620-626.

LOW BIRTHWEIGHT

Sarale E. Cohen, M.D.

*Both low birthweight infants and learning disabled children are
heterogeneous groups. On the average, low birthweight infants perform
slightly less well on various cognitive and behavioral tasks during childhood
than do infants of normal birthweight, but many perform at normal levels
or higher. Dr. Cohen suggests that future researchers assess particular
subgroups of low birthweight infants, such as infants born small for gestational age (rather than merely early) and those who have suffered intraventricular hemorrhages, and that they also subdivide outcomes instead of rely-
ing on global measures such as IQ.*

*Dr. Cohen reviews the literature on the association between low birth-
weight and learning disabilities or behaviors related to learning disabilities.
She also discusses the influence of social factors on the development of low
birthweight children. A disproportionate number of low birthweight babies
are born to mothers from lower social classes, and the question of whether
low social class compounds or masks deficits originally caused by low birthweight is still unanswered. A number of studies show that low social class
has a considerably more depressing effect on IQ and school performance
than low birthweight. However, children who are low in social class and
were also underweight at birth consistently score lower than other birthweight and social class groups.*

Low birthweight infants are studied frequently, as they are a prototypic
risk group and easily identified. About 7 percent of surviving infants are low

birthweight, making it the most common perinatal complication. Because low birthweight is considered a marker of fetal immaturity and of potential central nervous system insult, it has been hoped that the study of low birthweight infants will provide hypotheses as to underlying causes of brain dysfunction.

A number of review articles have summarized research on the development of the low birthweight infant (Caputo & Mandell 1970, Fitzhardinge 1976, Harper & Wiener 1965, Kopp in press, Kopp & Parmelee 1979). None has focused on learning disabilities though all have reported on many different outcomes. The consensus is that the low birthweight infant is at risk for a variety of intellectual, school, and behavioral tasks but that many low birthweight children do very well. The variability in performance that is always found spurs continued research.

Low birthweight, though easily defined as a birthweight less than 2,500 grams, is not actually a single variable. It includes both preterm infants (those born before 37 weeks of gestation) and small-for-gestational-age infants (SGAs), whether born early or at term. The SGA has different problems and different perinatal antecedent conditions than the low birthweight preterm infant whose weight is appropriate for gestational age.

In relating low birthweight to learning disabilities one must remember that learning disabled children, too, are a very heterogeneous group. In this paper, recent studies will be reviewed that examine the association between low birthweight and learning disabilities or behaviors related to learning disabilities: intelligence, school performance and reading, motor development, visual-motor integration, and behavioral/emotional problems.

The role of social factors in increasing the vulnerability of the low birthweight child will be considered as well. Studies of low birthweight children, though often overrepresenting disadvantaged backgrounds, include a range of social classes. The social class of a particular sample needs to be considered, because low birthweight and low social class are hopelessly confounded. In addition, social factors that are associated with low birthweight, such as ethnicity, prenatal care, and parental education, are also associated with the dependent measures used, such as intelligence and school achievement.

Intelligence

Although all studies report a wide range of intellectual outcomes for low birthweight subjects, in every study the mean score for low birthweight infants is lower than average. Nonetheless, the mean IQ is still within the normal range, according to most studies.

In a study by Drillien and colleagues (1980), IQ data for low birthweight and control groups were obtained for each of four social classes (middle to low). The data indicate clear birthweight differences as well as social class differences within each birthweight group. The low birthweight children scored worse than control children of the same social class. However, larger differences were found between social class groups than between birthweight groups (see Table 6).

Table 6. Intelligence Scores—by Birthweight and Social Class

	Social Class			
	Middle			Poor
Birthweight	1	2	3	4
Control	120	109	103	94
Low Birthweight	110	105	98	91

From: C. M. Drillien, A. J. M. Thomson, & K. Burgoyne, 1980. Low-birthweight children at early school-age: A longitudinal study. *Developmental Medicine and Child Neurology* 22:26-47.

In general, studies have shown an overreliance on a single composite score of intelligence to indicate dysfunction. Specific scores, rather than global scores, are now thought to be more useful at all ages. Thus, for example, the Bayley Scales have been divided into components such as vocal/social, eye-hand coordination, object relations, imitation, and manipulation in order to assess strengths and deficits in particular areas (Gaiter 1982, Siegel 1982).

School Performance and Reading

Many reports, both old and new, indicate a higher incidence of perceptual-motor problems, language problems, and other learning problems in low birthweight children (e.g., Parkinson, Wallis, & Harvey 1981, Caputo & Mandell 1970).

Failure in school or attendance in a special class was reported for 30 percent of low birthweight children with IQs over 100 and 36 percent of those with IQs over 90 (Fitzhardinge & Steven 1972). In a study of very low birthweight children, Hunt and colleagues (1982) calculated a similar "learning disability" rate: 37 percent, after dropping retarded children from the calculation.

Data from the Collaborative Perinatal Project pertinent to learning disabilities have been presented for a cohort of approximately 30,000 seven-year-olds (Nichols & Chen 1981). Children with IQs under 80 and those with serious neurological abnormalities such as cerebral palsy were excluded from the cohort. In the total group of 30,000, there were 2,499 children with learning difficulties. Among the 2,285 low birthweight children in the group, however, 251 were identified as learning disabled. Although 62 variables from the prenatal and perinatal period were examined, including low birthweight, most were not significantly associated with learning disabilities. Learning disabilities were strongly related to socioeconomic and demographic variables rather than to birth variables, although the risk was higher (1.3 times) for the low birthweight child.

The reading scores of low birthweight children tend to be slightly below average, but the difference is minimal and not found in all studies. For example, Kitchen and colleagues (1980) found no significant differences between low birthweight and full birthweight children in reading, and Drillien and colleagues (1980) reported lower reading scores only for the low birthweight group whose status was neurologically abnormal at one year.

Motor Development and Visual-Motor Integration

Low birthweight infants typically score lower on motor development both in infancy and in the preschool years than do infants in control groups. Furthermore, the motor scores are lower than the same infants' mental scores (Field et al. 1982, Hunt 1981, Taub, Goldstein, & Caputo 1977). The meaning of this lowered motor performance warrants examination. Knobloch and colleagues (1982) maintain that early motor abnormalities are an indication of problems in central nervous system integrity, and that an infant with minor or major motor abnormalities is at greater risk for learning or behavioral disabilities.

At school age, follow-up studies report tests primarily of visual-motor functioning, not motor behavior itself. Visual-motor integration is an area of behavior that has been a very consistent problem for the low birthweight child (Caputo & Mandell 1970, Drillien et al. 1980, Hunt, Tooley, & Harvin 1982). According to one investigator, impairment of visual experience may be the source of the somewhat lower intelligence test scores obtained in low birthweight children (Phillips 1968). Others speculate that the deficit in visual-motor integration is based on either subtle brain dysfunction or a limitation of brain cell growth to which the visual system may be particularly susceptible (Taub, Goldstein, & Caputo 1977). The results indicating impairment in the visual area have many implications for future research.

Behavioral/Emotional Problems

Behavioral and emotional problems have been much less studied than cognitive variables. Although an earlier review (Caputo & Mandell 1970) suggested that preterm infants have a higher incidence of deviant behavior, particularly disorganized, hyperkinetic, and maladaptive behavior, the evidence is somewhat equivocal. Some studies report an association between low birthweight and behavioral or emotional disturbance; others do not. The differences are due to methods, age at assessment, and amount of control for social class factors.

Escalona (1982) looked at emotional adjustment in the preschool years in low birthweight children. Extensive assessment, observations, and interviews were used to obtain measures of the child's adjustment starting at 15 months of age. The 27 children (from a total of 97) who at age 40 months were rated overtly maladjusted had lower developmental scores not only at 40 months but, when their records were examined retrospectively, as early as 15 months. The relationship between neurological measures and emotional adjustment was not tested. This study is an important addition to the research literature on the low birthweight child and provides new developmental data. Such data, potentially, can provide a clearer understanding of the antecedents of school problems.

As a group, then, low birthweight children function somewhat less competently than full-term, full birthweight children with comparable social backgrounds. In spite of normal IQ, the group is at risk for learning disabilities.

Several subgroups within the general low birthweight category are known or suspected to be at greater risk than the low birthweight average for gestational age. First, most (not all) studies show that small-for-gestational-age infants, whether born at term or before, have more intellectual, educational, and behavioral problems than do low birthweight children born early only (e.g., Neligan et al. 1976). A second potentially high-risk subgroup consists of low birthweight infants who have suffered intraventricular hemorrhage, though long-term data on this group have not been collected. Finally, what about the extremely low birthweight infant (1,000 grams or less), whose chances for survival have increased so greatly in recent years? This group, too, has not been studied for long enough to identify childhood consequences. School-age data on these infants will be of great interest.

Social Factors

One of the most widely recognized facts in the area of the development of the low birthweight child is the overwhelming role played by social factors. The confounding of social factors both with low birthweight itself and with the dependent measures used with low birthweight children has been noted in every comprehensive review of the development of the low birthweight child since 1940. Repeatedly, social factors have been shown to be the most reliable predictors of later outcome—which is not to say that biological risk factors are unimportant. What is the impact of the double disadvantage presented by adverse perinatal and social factors?

A number of investigators have written about the interaction of biological and social factors. Drillien's (1964) classic study of close to 600 premature infants, with prospective data up to age seven, reported that low birthweight children who came from disadvantaged social circumstances were more adversely affected than those who came from middle class homes. In contrast, Wiener and colleagues (1965) did not find that low birthweight children were particularly vulnerable to a bad environment. The recent study by Drillien and colleagues (1980) with a new cohort found that low birthweight children scored consistently lower than control children for each social class; however, the difference was greater in children from middle class homes for most measures. For example, the highest social class had a mean IQ of 120 for the control group and 110 for the low birthweight group, whereas the lowest social class had a mean IQ of 94 for the control group and 91 for the low birthweight group. The authors suggested that in lower class homes the effect of low birthweight was diminished by the effect of the adverse environment. There is no doubt that the lowest performing group in all studies is the group that is disadvantaged both socially and biologically.

In studying learning disabilities, the fact that regardless of biological risks, lower socioeconomic groups function at a lower level makes interpretation of dependent measures complex. Grotberg (1970) makes the point that we need to avoid an approach that sets a standard IQ criteria and excludes disadvantaged children who show symptoms of learning disabilities but whose problems may be masked by the overall lower test performance of children from poverty backgrounds.

Future Directions

This review has raised more questions than it has answered. Although there are some indications that low birthweight children are at increased risk for learning disabilities, the significant antecedent conditions are not known. Nor is it known why some children are vulnerable and some are not. The range of functioning that occurs, even in very low birthweight infants who have suffered a number of hazards, is astounding.

There are some intriguing hints in the research literature as to areas of problematic functioning, beginning in early infancy, that are ideal areas for continued research. One such area is sensory processing in infancy — which may be the analogue of information processing in the school-age child. In some studies of visual processing, preterm infants show less maturity than do full-term infants. One group of investigators has speculated that the relative immaturity of the visual system at birth makes it vulnerable to problems from exposure to visual stimulation before term date (Friedman, Jacobs, & Werthmann 1981). Korner (1981), however, suggested that the deficits may not be due to an insult to the immature system but rather that the preterm birth may have disrupted or slowed the maturation.

Neurophysiological data represent another source that has promise. Although it is fairly common to study neurophysiological functioning in low birthweight infants, additional neurophysiological data are rarely obtained during the school years. Also useful would be more detailed research on the specific environmental variables that may interact with biological factors to influence outcome for the low birthweight child. In addition to research in these and other areas, theoretical models that could be used to guide research and to integrate the existing empirical data are needed.

REFERENCES

Caputo, D. V., & Mandell, W. 1970. Consequences of low birthweight. *Developmental Psychology* 3:363-383.

Drillien, C. M. 1964. *The growth and development of the prematurely born infant.* Edinburgh: Livingstone.

Drillien, C. M., Thomson, A. J. M., & Burgoyne, K. 1980. Low-birth-weight children at early school-age: A longitudinal study. *Developmental Medicine and Child Neurology* 22:26-47.

Escalona, S. K. 1982. Babies at double hazard: Early development of infants at biologic and social risk. *Pediatrics* 70:670-676.

Field, T., Dempsey, J. R., Ting, G. T., Hallock, N., Dabiri, C., & Shuman, H. H. 1982. Respiratory distress syndrome: Perinatal prediction of one year development outcome. *Seminars in Perinatology* 6:288-293.

Fitzhardinge, P. M. 1976. Follow-up on the low birthweight infant. *Clinics in Perinatology* 3:503-516.

Fitzhardinge, P. M., & Steven, E. M. 1972. The small-for-date infant. II. Neurological and intellectual sequelae. *Pediatrics* 50:50-57.

Friedman, S. L., Jacobs, B. S., & Werthmann, M. W. 1981. Sensory processing in pre- and full-term infants in the neonatal period. In S. L. Friedman & M. Sigman (Eds.), *Preterm birth and psychological development.* New York: Academic Press.

Gaiter, J. L. 1982. The effects of intraventricular hemorrhage on Bayley developmental performance in preterm infants. *Seminars in Perinatology*

6:305-316.

Grotberg, E. 1970. Neurological aspects of learning disabilities: A case for the disadvantaged. *Journal of Learning Disabilities* 3:321-327.

Harper, P. A., & Wiener, G. 1965. Sequelae of low birthweight. *Annual Review of Medicine* 16:405-420.

Hunt, J. V. 1981. Predicting intellectual disorders in childhood for preterm infants with birthweights below 1501 gm. In S. L. Friedman & M. Sigman (Eds.), *Preterm birth and psychological development*. New York: Academic Press.

Hunt, J. V., Tooley, W. H., & Harvin, D. 1982. Learning disabilities in children with birthweights < 1500 grams. *Seminars in Perinatology* 6:280-287.

Kitchen, W. H., Ryan, M. M., Rickards, A., McDougall, A. B., Billson, F. A., Keir, E. H., & Naylor, F. D. 1980. A longitudinal study of very low-birthweight infants. IV. An overview of performance at eight years of age. *Developmental Medicine and Child Neurology* 22:172-188.

Knobloch, H., Malone, A., Ellison, P. H., Stevens, F., & Zdeb, M. 1982. Considerations in evaluating changes in outcome for infants weighing less than 1,501 grams. *Pediatrics* 69:285-295.

Kopp, C. B. In press. Risk factors in development. In P. Mussen (Ed.), *Manual of child psychology*, 4th ed. (Vol. II). New York: Wiley.

Kopp, C. B., & Parmelee, A. H. 1979. Prenatal and perinatal influences on infant behavior. In J. Osofsky (Ed.), *Handbook of infant development*. New York: Wiley.

Korner, A. F. 1981. Sensory responsiveness and social behavior in the neonatal period: A review of chapters 9 & 10. In S. L. Friedman & M. Sigman (Eds.), *Preterm birth and psychological development*. New York: Academic Press.

Neligan, G. A., Kolvin, I., Scott, D. Mc.I., & Garside, R. F. (Eds.). 1976. *Born too soon or born too small*. London: Spastics International Medical Publications.

Nichols, P. L., & Chen, T-C. 1981. *Minimal brain dysfunction: A prospective study*. Hillsdale, NJ: Erlbaum.

Parkinson, C. E., Wallis, S., & Harvey, D. 1981. School achievement and behavior of children who were small-for-dates at birth. *Developmental Medicine and Child Neurology* 23:41-50.

Phillips, C. J. 1968. The Illinois test of psycholinguistic abilities: A report on its use with English children and a comment on the psychological sequelae of low birthweight. *British Journal of Disorders in Children* 2-3:143-149.

Siegel, L. S. 1982. Reproductive, perinatal, and environmental variables as predictors of development of preterm (< 1501 grams) and full-term children at 5 years. *Seminars in Perinatology* 6:274-279.

Taub, H. B., Goldstein, K. M., & Caputo, D. V. 1977. Indices of prematurity as discriminators of development in middle childhood. *Child Development* 48:797-805.

Wallis, S. M., & Harvey, D. R. 1980. Small-for-date babies; their problems and their future. In B. A. Wharton (Ed.), *Topics for prenatal care.* London: Pitman Medical.

Wiener, G., Rider, R. V., Oppel, W. C., Fischer, L. K., & Harper, P. A. 1965. Correlates of low birthweight: Psychological status at six to seven years of age. *Pediatrics* 35:434-444.

ISSUES IN INFANT ASSESSMENT

Michael Lewis, Ph.D.
and Nathan Fox, Ph.D.

Most behavioral and physiological techniques now available for infant assessment are either known to be poor predictors of later performance or so new that their predictive power is still unknown. After reviewing these techniques, Drs. Lewis and Fox suggest that maximizing their predictive accuracy requires attention to several assessment issues.

First, Drs. Lewis and Fox recommend that researchers adopt an interactional model of development and attempt to include environmental variables (such as social class) in their study designs. Second, repeated assessments should be made, partly because environmental factors continue to interact with biological ones throughout life and partly because change is characteristic of human development. Third, as Dr. Cohen pointed out, children's capacities and skills should be measured specifically; two children with the same IQ may have very different profiles of particular abilities. Finally, Drs. Lewis and Fox outline a three-stage screening process that could be used as a model in attempting the early identification of infants and children with learning disabilities and other neurological problems.

Many behavioral and physiological measures are available for the assessment of early infant competence (see Table 7). Some, such as the Bayley Scales of Infant Development and the Brazelton Neonatal Assessment Scale, are good indicators of an infant's current status but poor predictors of later performance. Others show promise of greater predictive power but have been in use for only a short time, so that we cannot be sure. Infant visual attention, for example, is predictive of subsequent intellectual ability at least at age two (Lewis & Brooks-Gunn 1981, Lewis & Baldini 1979). Most electrophysiological techniques assessing subtle differences in brain functioning are also too new to have been used in longitudinal assessments. Some, such as the CAT scan and BEAM, seem able to distinguish between dyslexic and normal children of school age (Hier, LeMay, & Rosenberger 1978, Duffy et al. 1980), and many can identify abnormalities during infancy. However, it is uncertain which abnormalities in young infants might be correlated with learning disabilities if the infants were followed longitudinally into childhood.

Making the best use of the existing infant assessment techniques, and refining them to improve their predictive power, requires an understanding of some general issues in infant assessment. These include (1) models of development, (2) repeated assessment, (3) taxonomies of different skills, and (4) screening and follow-up assessments.

Table 7. Infant Assessment Techniques

Behavioral Techniques

Infant Intelligence Tests
  Bayley Scales of Infant Development
  Brunet-Lezine Test
  Cattell Infant Intelligence Scale
  Gesell Developmental Schedules
  Griffiths Scale of Mental Development
Brazelton Neonatal Assessment Scale
Measures of Infant Attention

Electrophysiological Techniques

Evoked Responses
  Somatosensory (SER)
  Visual (VER)
  Brainstem Auditory (BER)
Electroencephalogram (EEG)
Brain Electrical Activity Mapping (BEAM)
Computerized Axial Tomography (CAT scan)
Positron Emission Tomography (PET scanner)
Nuclear Magnetic Resonance (NMR)

Models of Development

The three main models of development can be characterized, in simple terms, as the biological, the environmental, and the interactional models (Lewis & Taft 1982). The biological model is based on the belief that the status of an infant at one point in time is predictive of the infant's status at a second point in time. It is assumed that biology alone controls capacities, and that these capacities manifest themselves in the same way at different ages. The environmental model, in contrast, assumes that the subsequent capacity of the child is best predicted from the nature of the environment. In this model, the child's environment accounts for the child's future status or capacity. The interactive model sees both the child's biological status and the environment as affecting future competence. Development is seen as an ongoing interaction between the organism and its environment. Thus, the child's future capacities will be determined by an interaction between earlier status variables and environmental variables.

The study of these three models and the data they have generated suggests that the interactional model perhaps best reflects the development process in both normal and learning disabled children. This fact has important implications for assessment. First, it suggests that any assessment procedure should not only measure the capacities of the child, however, one may wish to characterize them, but should measure aspects of the child's environment as well. Existing data seem to show that, regardless of how exact any particular infant assessment procedure may be, its power to predict later functioning will be improved if measures of the child's environment are also obtained and evaluated. For example, Broman and colleagues (1975) found that maternal education was a better predictor of preschool IQ than any medical or psychological variables recorded for either mother or child. However, as noted in the preceding paper (''Low Birthweight''by Sarale Cohen), the group that regularly scores lowest in studies is composed of low birthweight children from the lower social classes.

Second, an interactional model of development suggests a need for repeated assessments.

Repeated Assessments

In most cases, assessment is a one-time thing. For example, a newborn, after exhibiting a certain risk symptom, might be assessed for central nervous system dysfunction. Either the assessment demonstrates that the infant has a difficulty, or it shows that the infant does not. The assumption is that infants who do show dysfunction will continue to demonstrate it unless some intervention is initiated. Likewise, it is assumed that children who show no dysfunction will remain free of difficulties. Such an assumption, as we have indicated, is predicated on the notion that the existence (or absence) of a particular symptom of dysfunction will endure over time. While this is certainly the case for extreme dysfunctions, the data in general do not support this notion.

That manifestations of dysfunction may appear or disappear after an initial assessment can be taken to indicate either poor measurement techniques or changeable development on the part of the organism. Whichever interpretation one chooses, it should be clear that multiple assessments are necessary. For example, preterms over 1,500 grams are found even with corrected age to lag behind their term counterparts for the first year or two of life. However, by age two the preterm children appear equal to the term (Zarin-Ackerman & Lewis 1977). Such findings indicate that with repeated assessments it is possible to witness the decline of dysfunction in a particular subgroup. Equally likely is the appearance of a dysfunction not noted earlier. For example, cerebral palsied children often appear quite normal until six months of age or later, when they are unable to sit up.

Thus, while early examination might reveal normal development, some dysfunctions cannot be detected until a particular skill fails to emerge. This may hold true for language dysfunctions; that is, until normal language fails to appear, it may not be possible to discover that language function is impaired.

Multiple Skills

One of the major conceptual difficulties facing investigators of early development and subsequent dysfunction is the need to develop a taxonomy of skills or capacities. Although one might wish to characterize children in some overall way (for example, by IQ), it is apparent that children's capacities and skills are not neatly bundled. One of the failures of general IQ tests in infancy is that they do not reflect the variety of skills and competences that exist. Perhaps nowhere is this more obvious than in studies of children with learning disabilities and other perceptual or language disorders. These children have normal general cognitive ability, but at the same time certain skills and capacities are noticeably impaired.

A working taxonomy of such skills and capacities needs to be created. This task will not be easy, partly because of the discrepancies between our psychoeducational descriptions of competence and biological descriptions of the underlying mechanisms that may control these skills. Despite this problem (and others), it is essential that measurement of infants' abilities focus on patterns of specific behaviors and dysfunctions rather than on global variables.

Screening and Follow-Up Assessments

From a practical viewpoint, some problems of identification require only a single observation of dysfunction. In other cases, three levels of assessment are called for. The first level is essentially a screening procedure to divide children into three categories: certain, suspect, and nonsuspect. It is important, of course, to minimize the number of children placed in the wrong category. False negatives and false positives both present problems. For example, if a condition is to be corrected by surgery, then a false positive is of concern. If a treatment is not dangerous, expensive, or stigmatizing, then over-identifying may be preferable to under-identifying.

At the next level, those in the suspect category are assessed, using more complex procedures, to explore the extent and type of dysfunction that may be present. At the third level, information on the specific dysfunction is gathered for the purpose of intervention and treatment. At this level an assessment of the child's strengths and weaknesses can guide program placement and individualized interventions and provide a baseline against which to measure the child's progress.

At the primary level, a test only has to separate children into suspect, certain, and nonsuspect categories. Primary tests should be short. They should be designed for use in well baby clinics, pediatricians' offices, community health and hospital clinics, and perhaps the home. A variety of professionals should be able to administer these tests with a minimum of training.

At the secondary level, the function of a test is to provide more information on those children classified as suspect on the primary test. Although more detailed, the secondary test should be relatively easy to administer in a wide range of settings by many different personnel. This test should cover a variety of developmental domains, should include numerous skills within each domain, and should provide a profile of abilities by domain in order to pinpoint areas of dysfunction. Testing time would be longer, and scoring more complex, than for primary tests.

Finally, tertiary tests should be the most exact, and they require the most sophisticated measurement and technology. The assessment instruments shown in Table 7 are customarily used at this level of assessment, and it is at this level that causal relationships between infant deficits and childhood learning disabilities can potentially be established.

As we have tried to make clear, a fuller understanding of basic assessment issues should improve our ability to identify infants with early dysfunction and to predict—possibly even prevent—later negative outcomes.

REFERENCES

Broman, S. H., Nichols, P. L., & Kennedy, W. A. 1975. *Preschool IQ:*

Prenatal and early developmental correlates. Hillsdale, NJ: Erlbaum.

Duffy, F. H., Denckla, M. B., Bartels, P. H., & Sandini, G. 1980. Dyslexia: Regional differences in brain electrical activity by topographic mapping. *Annals of Neurology* 7:412-420.

Hier, D., LeMay, M., & Rosenberger, P. 1978. Developmental dyslexia. *Archives of Neurology* 35:90-92.

Lewis, M., & Baldini, N. 1979. Attentional processes and individual differences. In G. Hale & M. Lewis (Eds.), *Attention and cognitive development*. New York: Plenum.

Lewis, M., & Brooks-Gunn, J. 1981. Visual attention at three months as a predictor of cognitive functioning at two years of age. *Intelligence* 5:131-140.

Lewis, M., & Taft, L. T. (Eds.). 1982. *Developmental disabilities: Theory, assessment and intervention.* New York: S. P. Medical & Scientific Books.

Zarin-Ackerman, J., Lewis, M., & Driscoll, J. M. Jr. 1977. Language development in 2-year-old normal and risk infants. *Pediatrics* 59:982-986 (supplement).

PART II
FORUM

Editor's note

The forum portion of the Round Table was moderated by Frederick C. Robbins, M.D., President of the Institute of Medicine, National Academy of Sciences. In addition to Dr. Robbins, Dr. Larry Silver, and the authors of the papers summarized in Part I, the following individuals took part in the forum. Their full addresses appear in the list of participants and observers at the front of the book.

William L. Byrne, Ph.D., Professor of Biochemistry, University of Tennessee Center for Health Sciences

Lynne Cannon, Ph.D., ACLD Scientific Studies Committee

Charlotte Catz, M.D., Chief, Pregnancy and Perinatology Section, National Institute of Child Health and Human Development

Joseph S. Drage, M.D., Chief, Developmental Neurology Branch, National Institute of Neurological and Communicative Disorders and Stroke

Veronika E. Grimm, Ph.D., Director, Learning Disabilities Project, Weizmann Institute of Science (Israel)

Doris B. Haire, President, American Foundation for Maternal and Child Health

Barbara McElgunn, Chairman, Canadian ACLD Research and Information Committee

Audrey R. McMahon, ACLD Scientific Studies Committee and Symposium Coordinator

Shirley Post, Executive Director, Canadian Institute of Child Health

Joyce Riley, ACLD Scientific Studies Committee

John Wacker, Chairman, ACLD Scientific Studies Committee

Dr. Frederick Robbins, who served as moderator, began the discussion by comparing the authors of the papers summarized in Part I to the famous blind men who encountered an elephant. ''Groping to describe this beast with a very small portion of it at our command,'' he said, scientists from different disciplines and different backgrounds must search for ways to communicate.

He invited the participants to exchange ideas and drew their attention especially to several issues. First, he emphasized that the causes of learning disabilities are clearly many. Partly for that reason, those attempting to understand and prevent learning disabilities face problems of definition and taxonomy. In addition, the need to relate events that are distant in time (that is, perinatal events and behavior in the school-age child) creates difficulties both for scientific researchers and for those concerned with prevention and public health. Dr. Robbins asked the participants to respond to these issues, and to suggest an interdisciplinary research agenda for the future.

The discussion that followed centered on four main topics: definitional issues, the relevance (or lack thereof) of animal models to human behavior, the need to link biochemistry and behavior, and problems of prediction, prevention, and intervention.

DEFINITIONAL ISSUES

Incidence of Learning Disabilities

Early in the discussion, Dr. William Byrne asked a basic question. ''How many learning disabled children are there? What percentage of the children in the country belong to this group?''

Dr. Larry Silver replied that the incidence of learning disabilities depends on how they are defined. If one uses the definition that appears in Public Law 94-142,* Dr. Silver said, then 3 to 7 percent of the school population is probably affected — some three to ten million children. If one uses a definition

---

* The definition in Public Law 94-142, which specifies services for all handicapped school pupils, reads: ''The term 'children with specific learning disabilities' means those children who have a disorder in one or more of the basic psychological processes involved in understanding or in using language, spoken or written, which disorder may manifest itself in imperfect ability to listen, think, speak, read, write, spell, or do mathematical calculations. Such disorders include such conditions as perceptual handicaps, brain injury, minimal brain dysfunction, dyslexia, and developmental aphasia. Such term does not include children who have learning problems which are primarily the result of visual, hearing, or motor handicaps, of mental retardation, of emotional disturbance, or of environmental, cultural, or economic disadvantage'' (Federal Register 1977, quoted in Kirk & Kirk 1983).

that links learning disabilities more explicitly to central nervous system dysfunction, as the ACLD prefers, then the incidence might be slightly lower.

Today, many children who in the past might have been labeled slow learners or behavior problems are being diagnosed as learning disabled. For this reason, Dr. Silver continued, the incidence of learning disabilities appears to be increasing although, in fact, it may not be. He drew a parallel with the history of child abuse. During the first year after the term was introduced in the early 1960s, there was a tenfold increase in reported cases.

Dr. Silver also pointed out that learning disabilities are not limited to children. "Those of us who started looking at children with learning disabilities got older," he observed, "and we began writing about adolescents with learning disabilities. Now that we have more gray hair, we're writing about adults with learning disabilities." It is no longer generally believed that learning disabilities can be cured through remedial help. Although some children who are taught to build on strengths and develop effective learning strategies may learn to work around their disabilities and show no evidence of academic problems by sixth or seventh grade, others continue to show signs of learning disabilities at age 40, 50, or 60.

Dr. Vernonika Grimm asked Dr. Silver whether the incidence of learning disabilities varies from one country to another. Dr. Silver replied that differences among languages may affect incidence. In the 1970s, he said, one researcher studying a population of Japanese children said they had virtually no reading difficulties; the concrete graphics of the Japanese language were thought to explain this finding. Later researchers obtained different results, reporting roughly the same incidence of reading problems in Japan as in this country. However, it is still thought that learning disabilities are less common in children whose languages use very concrete symbols than in children whose languages use abstract and visually similar symbols such as d, b, p, and q.

Lumpers and Splitters

Dr. Silver suggested that those concerned with defining learning disabilities can be classified as "lumpers" or "splitters." The lumpers place disabilities in large groups and use familiar terms such as dyslexia (reading disability), dyscalculia (math disability), and dysgraphia (written language disability). The splitters would say that a term like dyslexia is descriptive, not diagnostic. They want to break down reading difficulties into specific areas of dysfunction. "Dyslexia means that the child can't read, but it does not say why. To a splitter, it would seem more useful to say that the child cannot read because of specific problems with perception, sequencing, memory, and so on," Dr. Silver concluded.

Several participants agreed that splitting is preferable to lumping. Dr. John Sever pointed out that, far from splitting learning disabled children into more precisely defined groups, educators and physicians often lump them with children who are mentally retarded. Dr. Hugo Moser said splitting should take priority over lumping because learning disabilities are not a single entity.

Dr. Robbins summed up: "I don't think we should apologize for being splitters, because that's the way science moves. You have to split before you can lump, and there's no point in lumping before you've done the appropriate splitting."

If It's Environmentally Caused, Is It a Learning Disability?

The representatives of the American and Canadian ACLDs who attended the Round Table had no doubt about the answer to this basic definitional question: an unequivocal no. As John Wacker explained, these organizations define learning disabilities as stemming from identifiable or inferred central nervous system dysfunction. Thus, if the source of a child's difficulties is social, educational, or environmental, the child may have a learning problem or a learning difficulty but not a learning disability.

Dr. Robbins asked the participants whether they were prepared to agree that learning disabilities necessarily reflect a disturbance or dysfunction in central nervous system functioning rather than a disturbance in social functioning or some other environmental area. Their replies seemed to show a great interest in researching central nervous system dysfunction as it relates to learning disabilities but a reluctance either to rule out social and environmental factors by definition or to ignore them. Both practically and theoretically, they seemed to feel, it is impossible to separate biological and environmental factors with precision, and perhaps simplistic to try.

Dr. Herbert Needleman led off with the comment that coming down firmly on either side of the biology-environment argument might stigmatize learning disabled children or their parents.

> I am certainly in great sympathy with mothers who have been
> led to feel guilty because they were told there was some social
> interaction that was compromising their child's behavior. As a
> psychiatrist, I encounter people with guilt because they have been
> told that somehow some aberrant interaction between them and
> their child has led to the disordered behavior, and that's a ter-
> ribly difficult thing to bear. On the other hand, it appears that a
> great many poor and minority children are labeled retarded,

learning disabled, or behaviorally disordered at school. Many of these children have linguistic problems but not neurological damage. If learning disabilities are assumed to reflect only CNS dysfunction, this could be used against some children. They need protection from a stigma of a different kind.

Dr. Moser continued, "The problem is that it's easy to say we won't call it a learning disability unless social problems are eliminated, but the act of eliminating them is very complicated." He offered the example of Spanish-speaking children in an English-speaking elementary school. "We cannot attribute their reading and writing problems to central nervous system abnormalities — though neither can we be sure that no such abnormalities are present," he said.

Dr. Sarale Cohen commented that in her work with low birthweight infants she sees a number of children with school problems from Spanish-speaking families. "If the children do have some kind of central nervous system insult," she said, "the insult is being masked by social factors at least up through age five and perhaps for several more years. We really have no way of knowing, because their performance on the measures we have available is depressed by social and cultural factors."

There may be an interaction between retardation of brain development and sociocultural factors, Dr. Joseph Altman added. "It is quite conceivable that a child could have a nervous system dysfunction that would be manifested as a learning disability only under certain circumstances," perhaps in a poverty environment where effective remedial measures were not available.

Barbara McElgunn reiterated the Canadian ACLD position, stating that her organization understood the difficulty of being certain about the source of a child's problems but adopted a definition specifying CNS dysfunction if the problems are to be called learning disabilities. One of the reasons for this, she continued, was that the organization wanted to increase professional and public awareness of the neurological basis of learning disabilities. "We want basic neurophysiological research on children," stated Dr. William Byrne.

Dr. Robbins replied that he was sympathetic to this position but felt that ruling out social factors "sets up an artificial system." A definition specifying CNS damage may be useful to some investigators, he went on, but there are problems with it. "First, you cannot rule out all socioeconomic factors — it's not possible. Second, some such factors may have effects that mimic learning disabilities caused by CNS damage. Third, in the last analysis, anything that happens to an organism is reflected in some biochemical event."

Dr. Bruce McEwen said that a distinction between "biochemical" and "environmental" causes of behavior seemed artificial to him, too. The example of stress, he said, shows that a specific mechanism can link chemical factors, including hormones that can lead to brain malformation, with environmental factors.

> If you grant that socioeconomic deprivation can result in stress, then many poverty children may be growing up with elevated levels of glucocorticoids around the clock. If glucocorticoids can inhibit brain cell division, including the microneurons that Dr. Altman discussed in his paper, then you have a very clear mechanism by which something environmental can directly affect brain structure and function.

He also discussed prenatal drugs, which are environmental influences on the fetus even though the damage done by them may be biochemical or neurological. "Various environmental factors," Dr. McEwen concluded, "could be influencing the actual chemical functioning of neurons as well as morphology."

Dr. Altman observed that it is quite possible for a variety of factors to have the same outcome. Dr. Artemis Simopoulos suggested dwarfism as an example. It can be caused organically, by a growth hormone deficiency, she said, but psychosocial deprivation can also interfere with growth. The effects of psychosocial dwarfism on linear growth are just the same as those of growth hormone deficiency, and both types of dwarfism are of interest to scientists who study nutrition.

"If there is anything that a developmental scientist can add to this discussion," said Dr. Michael Lewis,

> it is the fact that biological insult interacts with the nature of the environment in producing an outcome. As Dr. Altman said, the possibility that some biological perturbations may not manifest themselves unless the environment acts in a particular manner must be considered. Plasticity of structure and function is a hallmark of the central nervous system. It is neither abnormal nor unusual but instead is part of the nature of the human organism. Rather than try to work around environmental interactions, perhaps we need to think of models that would build these interactions into our assessment methods.

Dr. Grimm brought the discussion of definitional issues to a close by pointing out that researchers studying human problems are often forced to proceed without a clear understanding of whether the causes of the problems are biological, environmental, or both. Depression, schizophrenia, and other mental disorders, for example, deserve and receive much research attention despite confusion on this matter. "The ambiguities do not prevent neuroscientists from making the basic assumption that the brain in one way or another is the major organ involved," she said. "I think probably scientists studying learning disabilities can make the same assumption."

ANIMAL MODELS AND HUMAN BEHAVIOR

Much research on perinatal risk factors has been performed on animals (rodents, usually) rather than on human subjects as the papers summarized in Part I indicate. Dr. Simopoulos pointed out, however, that the natural physiological and behavioral patterns of different species vary greatly. She illustrated her point by quoting Gibbs and Seitchik (1980):

> Although unproved in humans, protein-calorie restriction in animals, particularly rodents, will result in neonates with fewer cells in many organs, particularly brain, and these animals will manifest learning disabilities if they survive. Contrariwise, the black bear gestates, delivers, and nurtures her cub during a prolonged period of total starvation. Applying the results of animal experiments, particularly those obtained in species where pregnancies are characterized by brief duration and large litters, to those of human beings may be illogical...

Dr. Altman pointed out that before Darwin showed the evolutionary continuity between animals and human beings, animal studies were not considered relevant to human behavior at all, because human beings were thought of as totally different creatures from animals. "Then animal models became fashionable, and there was a time in the 1920s when animal studies were believed to represent the scientific approach to all human problems. We seem to go through cycles. Today, you hear more and more people questioning the relevance of animal work."

How relevant are animal models to human behavior? When is it safe to assume that principles demonstrated in animal experiments also hold for human beings? These questions held great interest for the Round Table participants.

Timing: Rats Develop Faster

Dr. Ann Streissguth, whose ongoing Pregnancy and Health Study was described in her paper, works with human rather than animal subjects. However, she expressed enthusiasm for animal research, both as a source of leads and because "longitudinal" studies of rodents take so much less time than longitudinal studies of infants and children. "One reason I enjoy doing work on the effects of alcohol is that there is such an active animal literature to interact with," she said. "The outcome variables we are studying have at all points been tied as closely as possible to what we've learned from the animal literature, because with animals one can perform experiments that just can't be done on human beings, particularly in terms of brain studies." For example, she added, research showing hippocampal lesions in rats exposed to alcohol before birth has led her to develop behavioral tests for hippocampal function in humans to use in her study.

One reason that rats and mice are good experimental subjects for research on perinatal events, said Dr. McEwen, is that they are born in a state of neurological immaturity. As explained in Dr. Altman's paper, the nervous system of a rodent is much less fully developed at birth than that of a newborn primate or even guinea pig. In terms of sexual differentiation, Dr. McEwen said, the newborn rat is roughly as mature as the human fetus at midgestation. Therefore, one can study the effects of experimental manipulations on newborn rats that in primates would have to be studied in utero.

The chronology of neuron production in rodents has been carefully studied and is very systematic, Dr. Altman added. Neurons are produced in a precise sequence, one type on one day and another on another day. A trauma such as malnutrition, experienced by the pregnant rat on a particular day, affects the multiplication of cells programmed to form in the fetal brain on that day, and the loss is likely to be permanent. Parallel deficits may occur in human fetuses subjected to trauma for only a limited period of time. Dr. Simopoulos agreed that such findings are suggestive, though she reminded the group that the sequence of events in the development of the human brain is not so clearly defined.

Behavior: Rats Can't Read

Responding to the general question of animal models and their relevance to the study of learning disabilities, Dr. Needleman made an important point.

> The critical discriminator between animals and humans is not the use of tools, since some animals do use tools. The discriminator is the use of language. Despite the power of animal studies as aids in understanding physiological mechanisms (for instance), the inability of animals to use language places finite and permanent limits on their usefulness in understanding learning disabilities.

Even though some animals communicate, Dr. Simopoulos added, and some chimpanzees have been trained to use sign language, there are significant differences between animal communication and human language. "Therefore," she said, "we ought to be extremely careful about extrapolating from animal studies to human beings when it comes to language." Dr. Altman agreed. "Rats are good models for attentional behavior and spatial reasoning," he said, as their maze-learning abilities indicate. "But language use is something different. It involves symbols."

"From my research," Dr. Broman said, "it looks as if learning disabilities can be equated with poor linguistic abilities. I agree that characteristics associated with linguistic deficits in learning disabled children, such as attention and behavioral deficits, can be studied in animals. However, as Dr. Lewis pointed out in his paper, linguistic abilities themselves appear late. This affects both the issue of early screening and the issue of animal models." It would be especially useful, Dr. Broman added, if physiological research could provide clues to the reasons behind the commonly observed sex ratio of three or four learning disabled boys for every one learning disabled girl.

Dr. Lewis was dubious about animal models, in part because they often focus on phsysiology rather than on behavior.

> We have to make sure that the phenomena we're studying come as close as possible to what we're trying to understand in human children. Learning disabilities are not large behavioral changes caused by severe structural perturbation. They are very subtle behaviors in a human being who can do most everything but read.
>
> How similar in structure and function are a rat's brain, a pig's, a human's? If there are significant differences that relate to higher mental functioning, then our models must reflect this. I think it is important to focus more upon the behavioral outcome if, in fact, we wish to extend animal models to humans.

A difficulty with direct behavioral studies of animals, Dr. Sever said, is that behavioral assessments sometimes fail to pick up serious brain damage caused by infections or drugs. Drug research with primates has demonstrated that the brain of a monkey can sustain an alarming amount of damage that is undetectable on behavioral tests. "In our laboratory," Dr. Sever went on, "we can use Venezuelan encephalitis to produce severe hydrocephalus in 100 percent of our newborn monkeys. Nevertheless, these animals often function very normally." Using behavioral tests is fine if you do find an effect, Dr. Sever asserted, "but I would be reluctant to use a strictly behavioral approach in attempting, say, to screen for drugs that might produce subtle brain damage."

Similar observations have been reported concerning patients who have had frontal lobotomies, Dr. Needleman said. These patients seemed normal because they were not being tested for higher-order functions such as abstract reasoning — which can never be tested in infrahuman animals if they are normally absent. "Animal studies give rich and marvelously exciting information about lower-level mechanisms that form a substrate for behavior," Dr. Needleman concluded, "but in my opinion they cannot be translated without error to the functioning of children."

Dr. Sumner Yaffe suggested that greater efforts be made in the future to validate findings from animal research in studies with human subjects. "Part of the problem with animal models," he noted, "is that researchers trying to construct them usually spend their entire professional lives studying the animal species in question and never get around to studying humans. It is the old forest and trees story."

The Fundamental Nature of the Cell

Dr. McEwen admitted that he approached the study of the human being through the rat "with great trepidation." The cerebral cortex of the rat and the cerebral cortex of the human being are quite different in sophistication of organization. "A basic tenet certainly of the area I represent," Dr. McEwen said, "is that it is at the level of biochemical and cellular events that the human and rodent brain are likely to be most similar. The farther out you go in terms of behavior, the more dangerous extrapolations become, because you compound all the differences in neuroanatomical organization and phylogeny."

"I personally have to keep coming back to the fact that biology is unitary," said Dr. Robbins. "There is one biology, and if we understand it well enough then we can draw analogies accurately."

LINKING BIOCHEMISTRY AND BEHAVIOR

"I think the reason we got stuck on animal models," Dr. Lewis offered, "is that we are talking about the need to find some correspondence between what we call biological events and what we call behavioral events. Obviously, though, they are not independent."

In discussing this provocative idea, the participants concentrated on two points. First, because of new techniques for the direct study of the brain, information about brain structure and function that in the past would have been obtainable only through biological research with animals can now be gained by studying the living human brain. Second, scientists who study biology (especially in animals) and those who study behavior (especially in human beings) are making some progress in learning to communicate.

New Techniques for Studying the Human Brain

Modern scanning techniques, Dr. Moser began, give scientists an unprecedented opportunity to correlate human brain structure and function with behavior. "I'm particularly excited about the nuclear magnetic resonance (NMR) technique, because there is every reason to believe that it will not be harmful to the child. NMR, and positron emission tomography (the PET scanner) too, have the potential for allowing the study of chemical events as well as structural events. These techniques will eventually permit brain-behavior correlations that have never before been possible."

Dr. Silver agreed that NMR systems will be safer for children than the present PET scanner, which physicians try to avoid using on patients under age seventeen or so because of the radiation level it entails. However, he went on, early PET scanner research with adults has yielded some fascinating data.

> PET scans of schizophrenics show that their occipital cortexes do not shut down when they are asleep, as those of normal people do. PET (and CAT) scans are also being used to study a group of autistic children who have now reached their twenties, thirties, and forties. In the next five or ten years, I think NMR and the PET scanner are going to provide some extremely interesting information on how people learn — and, we hope, on why people have trouble learning.

"We know very little about the mechanisms of so-called normal learning," said Dr. Broman, "and this has implications for our ability to identify mechanisms in non-normal children. In the Developmental Neurology Branch of NINCDS, we have a program now asking for research on neurophysiological correlates of learning handicaps and , frankly, I am just as interested in seeing the data from the control subjects as the data from the learning handicapped group."

Dr. Sever asked whether anyone in the group knew of current studies involving PET or CAT scans of patients with learning disabilities. He said he knew of none, though in his own laboratory he is using PET and CAT scans on patients with amyotrophic lateral sclerosis, and some children with learning disabilities might be included in groups being studied for this or other reasons.

The CAT scan, Dr. Lewis pointed out, has been used in a number of studies comparing dyslexic and nondyslexic children. This technique is the source of information cited in Dr. McEwen's paper concerning the reversed asymmetry in the brains of many dyslexics. Although this asymmetry and dyslexia may be related, Dr. Lewis continued, there are no studies that have uncovered these neuroanatomic irregularities in infants and correlated them with later mental performance, since it would not be safe to use the scan to screen infants who do not have very definite problems.

Very low birthweight infants who have suffered intraventricular hemorrhage sometimes receive CAT scans, however. They are helpful in evaluating the severity of the hemorrhage, Dr. Lewis said, and some recent studies have shown correlations between the severity of the hemorrhage as measured by CAT scan and subsequent mental outcome. Dr. Cohen commented that long-term developmental data have not been collected as yet. In some studies the severity of neonatal brain hemorrhage was not associated with developmental problems as much as was the presence of neonatal illness. Existing data suggest that even in infants with neurophysiological evidence of severe brain insult there is much recovery. Dr. Joseph Drage added that ultrasound is also useful in identifying hemorrhages and their consequences in tiny infants.

Dr. Drage went on to point out that only a few neuroanatomical studies of the brains of deceased learning disabled children have been done, as noted in Dr. Moser's paper. "After some problems have been identified with the PET scanner and NMR," he suggested, "it might be useful to research these problems further through autopsy." Barbara McElgunn mentioned that scientists at the Canadian Brain Tissue Bank have expressed an interest in studying tissue samples from learning disabled persons. Audrey McMahon pointed out that a similar brain bank also exists in the United States. It was established by the Orton Dyslexia Society at the Beth Israel Hospital in Boston, and the work is supervised by Dr. A.M. Galaburda.

Interdisciplinary Communication and Training

"I feel like a bit of an apologist for the behavioral sciences," Dr. Lewis commented.

> Without denying that a great deal can be learned through neurophysiological and neuroanatomical research, we need to acknowledge the well-known scientific phenomenon that different measures often give different results. If we are truly interested in understanding basic relationships between brain structure and function and behavior, and also in identifying dysfunctional infants and children, then we are going to have to pay some attention to behavior, too, as we try to link these things together.

"Unfortunately," Dr. Robbins remarked bluntly, "the people making measurements in biology often don't know anything about behavior." Dr. McEwen elaborated:

> A problem that must be overcome is to convince people who have

a good grounding in basic neuroscience or biochemistry that behavioral research, despite its apparent deficiencies in quantitative precision and such, is scientifically respectable and does not deserve the degree of prejudice sometimes shown toward it. Speaking as a cell biologist who has spent sixteen years working in a behavioral sciences group, I can say that there is very beautiful, careful, rigorous, and interesting behavioral work being done. The exchange of information taking place at this conference bodes well for the future, but there is still this problem of prejudice to overcome.

Dr. Yaffe said that the National Institute of Child Health and Human Development is interested in moving biological and behavioral scientists closer together, and that a training program aimed at persuading biologists to study behavior is being planned. Dr. Sever added that he has been impressed with the interest in behavior shown by the field of obstetrics and gynecology in recent years. "The new subspecialty of maternal-fetal medicine could be important to people interested in learning disabilities," he observed.

What the study of learning disabilities requires, said Dr. Silver, "is the type of multidisciplinary research that various fields of medicine have gotten into in working on multifactorial illnesses such as hypertension." Like biological and behavioral scientists, he went on, research psychologists and clinicians often seem to live in different worlds. One of the goals of the National Institute of Mental Health is to further collaborative research by these groups, and they have recently tried to do this by developing an innovative training program.

First we took a group of people with clinical training — child psychiatrists — and gave them a one- or two-year fellowship for basic research. Then we chose a group of developmental psychologists who usually do research and put them through a one- or two-year clinical program. In this way, we hope to stimulate clinical research — and also to provide a sort of role model for the next generation on the matter of collaborative research.

"Some of my best friends are basic scientists and do research," confessed Dr. Don Creevy.

I've even done some basic research myself. But I'm a clinician, and I think the kind of training you're talking about has to begin in medical school and continue during residencies in obstetrics and gynecology. Quite frankly, I don't think obstetricians have a great deal of interest in the ultimate results of their work — in its possible effects on the school-age child, for instance. Their training simply doesn't prepare them to consider such things. In looking at the literature on learning disabilities, I'm astonished at how little of it appears in obstetrical journals. Our articles are all about anoxia, forceps trauma, immediate sequelae, that sort of thing.

"One of the things I would find valuable for the future," Dr. Streissguth contributed, "would be for those of us who do research to have more input from people actually dealing with learning disabled children." She explained that it is crucial in doing longitudinal work with children to select the right outcome variables for assessment at different ages. "We can only test our seven-year-olds once, for a couple of hours each," she said. "If we choose the wrong variables to study, an enormous opportunity will be lost."

Dr. Broman responded that age seven may be a little early to test for learning disabilities, because school performance is probably not stable at that time. In the Collaborative Perinatal Project, some children were identified as learning disabled at age seven. "We would have liked to assess these children again at nine or ten but were not able to do so," Dr. Broman said. Dr. Streissguth replied that this was very useful information, since her project hopes to provide for assessment at ages ten and thirteen as well as at seven.

Even with better training, communication, and techniques, Dr. Moser remarked, attempting to correlate brain and behavioral events, as Dr. Altman has in developing the animal model described in his paper, is a formidable challenge. "The only thing I have to say," Dr. Altman replied, "is that those of us who work with animals and those of us who work with children should listen to each other more. We're all engaged in the same enterprise, and I think we have to work together."

PREDICTION, PREVENTION, AND INTERVENTION

"Since the focus of this meeting is upon prenatal and perinatal factors that might relate to learning disabilities," said Dr. Yaffe, "what we need to develop is the ability to come into the hospital nursery and identify those infants who are at risk, whether for genetic reasons, environmental reasons, or both. This would permit early intervention."

Dr. Creevy agreed. "As a result of my review of the literature and listening to other speakers," he said, "I've been very impressed with the desirability of being able to identify the future learning disabled child at birth. If we could do that, and start remediation as soon as possible, it would be very, very helpful."

Prediction Problems and Research Needs

But, Dr. Lewis pointed out, not all difficulties are detectable at birth — which is only one of the problems involved in trying to predict learning disabilities in advance of their appearance at school age.

> We are capable at present of identifying many more children who are at serious risk for subsequent dysfunction at much earlier ages than we used to be. However, the development process is such that various behaviors emerge and fade out over time. There exists a set of complex behaviors in the seven-year-old that the newborn simply does not show. That is, while the underlying process might be the same, the behaviors are not. How can we say that a newborn, or a one-year-old, will have reading problems until we discover the precursors of reading that might reside in the infant? The problem, in a sense, is how to get from the things the newborn shows to those other, later kinds of behavior.

Dr. Robbins pointed out that even with a toxin or an infection that is known to cause prenatal damage, it is hard to be sure except in flagrant cases that a child's disability at age seven reflects that damage. "And, as Dr. Lewis said earlier, we're not talking about the flagrant. We're talking about some very subtle learning problems."

"I would concur with that," Dr. Yaffe said, "and I agree that there may be some predictive events that just don't take place until after the newborn period. But others will be evident at birth, and that's a nice time to be able to look. The hospital nursery represents a captive environment for most infants in this country, at least briefly."

Dr. Simopoulos suggested neonatal head circumference as one of the better predictors of later cognitive performance, particularly in low birthweight babies whose growth begins to slow before 26 weeks of gestation. These infants can now be identified through the use of ultrasound.

> According to a study by Harvey and others, which I cite in my paper, it appears that low birthweight infants who manifest fetal growth retardation prior to 26 weeks gestation had significantly lower scores for the general cognitive index than control children. This did not occur in children whose head growth began to slow later in gestation. The authors of the study concluded that prolonged slow growth in utero affects a child's later development and abilities, particularly performance and motor ability. Furthermore, these findings indicate that it is possible to predict at birth, on the basis of intrauterine ultrasonic growth patterns alone, those small-for-gestational-age newborns who are most

likely to have problems later.

Dr. Broman added that current studies of learning disorders, mental retardation, and intellectual performance in childhood at the NINCDS Development Neurology Branch show that head circumference at birth is a more efficient predictor than birthweight.

However, Dr. Broman went on, even head circumference at birth does not consistently predict learning problems if one requires children in the sample to have IQs of at least 90. "Neonatal size variables seem to be related to general cognitive ability but not to poor academic achievement in children of average intelligence," she said.

"As you all know," Dr. Cohen said, "there is a very high correlation between IQ and school achievement. That is the reason investigators of learning disabilities, who need to identify children whose achievement is noticeably lower than would be expected from their IQs, have to establish IQ cut-off points in looking at relationships between risk factors and disabilities."

Dr. Cohen also pointed out that when Lipper and colleagues stated that they could identify at birth those children most likely to have school problems, they were talking about group data.

> They do not talk about individual prediction and individual hit rates. I think there has to be a lot more emphasis on understanding what happens to individual children. In spite of the risk that low birthweight and low head circumference represent, I'm struck by the fact that so many children in these groups do function adequately. Group differences give us clues and hypotheses about the processes and risk factors that are operating, but they do not tell us about individual children. One of the things I would like to see studied more is compensatory mechanisms that might occur. Another is learning strategies in very young children and the environmental supports for those strategies.

Methodologically, Dr. Lewis said, a serious problem with developmental research is that Variable A (a perinatal event, say) may, in fact, be related to Variable B (a school performance measure, say) even though individual stability on these variables is lacking. A positive correlation between variables requires that the subjects in a sample maintain their relative positions on the two variables. "There is no way to demonstrate a relationship over time between A and B except through individual stability vis-a-vis the group," Dr. Lewis said.

He used crawling and walking as a simple example of two behaviors that appear to be related although they are not statistically correlated. "Some children learn to crawl earlier than others, but these children do not necessarily learn to stand or walk earlier. Thus, we cannot predict delayed walking from delayed crawling. This is a very standard problem in developmental science.''

Nonetheless, Dr. Lewis went on, if researchers wish to focus on a particular age,

> then I think there are certain categories of behavior or performance that should be investigated intensively. For the very young infant or newborn, the first such category is attention. Reliable and easily obtained measures of visual and auditory attention are available that potentially can even be used in clinical settings. As indicated in my paper, some measures of attention are correlated with cognitive performance at age two. The second candidate is intersensory integration—the ability of the young organism's nervous system to take data from two sensory modalities and integrate them into a coherent whole. The third is lateralization and differentiation within the central nervous system, at least at the level of the hemispheres.
>
> It seems clear to me that in order to understand structure, function, and behavior, we're going to have to commit ourselves ultimately to a matrix system in which different structures, functions, and behaviors interact in some very complex fashion. Therefore, we are going to have to commit ourselves to a set of dependent variables rather than a single one (such as IQ). However, a set of variables will generate an erratic profile which is not based on error variance. In other words, we will find that a child does well in one area and not well in another, but this will not mean that we have measured the child's abilities poorly. It will mean that various interactions generate this sort of uneven profile. The appeal I would make, as I did earlier, is that in developing our matrix we focus more on the behavioral aspects of dysfunction.

A matrix based on the approach of physiology, Dr. Moser suggested, might begin with three intersecting areas: behavior, etiology, and localization. Dr. Needleman suggested an alternate scheme involving four categories. ''The first would be phenotypic behavior, what you see the child doing, and that requires behavior analysis. Second, what functional disturbances can one measure and discriminate? That requires biochemistry, and bringing the child to the behavioral laboratory for testing. The third category would be etiological classifications, and the fourth would be response to therapy.'' Dr. Silver said that he would add a fifth variable, the temporal one. ''As Dr. Lewis observed in his paper, in studying learning disabled children, a single assessment is often not sufficient.''

"But even after only one assessment, if several are not possible, I think one should be prepared to do some intervention," Dr. Broman commented. "In my opinion, we know enough about modifying behavioral responses and improving learning rates or learning capacity to intervene on that level if not on a primary etiological level."

Prevention: The Smallpox Parallel

A conference like the present one has two products, Dr. Silver observed. One is an agenda for basic research that will allow development of the sort of matrixes just proposed, and the other is an agenda for public health. "The basic public health questions," he said, "are what do we already know and what can we do about it."

From the standpoint of basic research, Dr. Robbins commented, a concern with individual predictions is important. "From a public health standpoint, however, if there are ways to affect the overall statistical outcome for a risk group, they should be used."

After acknowledging that ways to do this may be hard to find until learning disabilities and their etiology are better understood, he offered a reassuring bit of medical history.

> I want to remind you that probably the greatest preventive measure ever developed was devised in the total absence of the basic science underlying it, namely, smallpox vaccination. Jenner did not even know there were such things as viruses. He had no concept of infectious disease, and yet he developed a very effective means of prevention. Now we have eliminated that disease (admittedly after many years) — and we still don't understand all the facts about it.

Dr. Robbins asked Dr. Cohen whether the low birthweight infant might represent an opportunity to follow the Jenner model. Since low birthweight is associated with cognitive deficits, reducing the incidence of low birthweight might reduce the incidence of deficits even though neither the reasons for infants' small size nor its connection with later disabilities were well understood.

"Certainly," Dr. Cohen replied.

> One thing that has been said in all the medical journals is that if we can prevent prematurity and low birthweight, we will have gone a long way toward preventing certain deleterious outcomes. However, we will probably get more payoff if we can separate low birthweight infants into subgroups. We must remember that

the risk for the group as a whole is only slightly higher than that for full birthweight infants.

"Would you comment on the relationship between maternal infection and low birthweight, Dr. Sever?" asked Dr. Robbins. "In addition to the infections covered in my paper," Dr. Sever answered, "there is evidence that mycoplasma, urinary tract infections, and chlamydia may cause low birthweight and damage to the child. It is possible that learning disabilities should be considered as one potential outcome."

Dr. Robbins said that the National Academy of Sciences and other funding agencies are eager not only to promote public health but to encourage basic research on such questions. For example, NICHD is holding a planning workshop on intrauterine growth retardation to pinpoint areas for further research. Drawing another medical analogy, Dr. Robbins said that without basic research on polio, "we could still be refining the respirator. In the long run, that is not the way to go."

Dr. Needleman commented that he recently read an article by Julius Comroe describing ten or twelve times when highly placed experts in medical science were very wrong, and two were in the field of polio vaccination. First, in 1930, one informed researcher said that polio vaccine was right around the corner. Then, around 1950, another expert said that developing a vaccine would require some 30 additional years of basic research. "It is quite clear that we do not need to know everything before we can develop appropriate remedies," Dr. Needleman said.

Some Practical Recommendations

"Part of the task of this group," Dr. Robbins said, "is to make recommendations that could be implemented now. Certain things are already known that should make it possible to reduce disabilities, including learning disabilities, in children. We've already discussed the advantages of reducing the incidence of prematurity and low birthweight. What other recommendations can we make?"

Dr. Creevy replied that in listening to the papers and discussion at the Round Table he had been impressed with how much scientists do know about the effects of some perinatal events and interventions on the infant or child. However, he went on,

> somewhere in my training I imprinted on the phrase, "Above all, do no harm," and I haven't had any reason to change my adherence to that principle in the time I've been practicing. I have spent the 22 years since I got out of medical school dumbfounded by the ignorance that we have of the techniques we use. It's as

if there were a large learning disability within the field of physicians who treat pregnant and laboring women. I even see an analogy between this behavior and the more serious and widespread learning disability that may be leading the human race toward nuclear destruction. So perhaps an intervention that this group could recommend would be a return to first principles. We should question more seriously whether we should be doing some of the things that we are doing, the results of which we don't really understand. That's basic public health, I think.

Joyce Riley commented that some intervention programs for learning disabled children, such as the use of stimulants, apparently do fall into the harmful category, and the participants seemed to agree. Dr. Silver pointed out, however, that stimulants have usually been prescribed for the hyperactivity and distractibility that often accompany learning disabilities rather than for learning disabilities themselves. "To me it doesn't mean much when a follow-up study says we took twenty children who couldn't read, put them on stimulants for a year, and found they still couldn't read."

"In addition to the principle that we must do no harm," said Dr. Moser, "implementation of what we know we should do is very important." Dr. Robbins suggested it might be possible right now to write a reasonable prescription that would reduce learning disabilities. It would specify, for example, good obstetrical care throughout pregnancy, a nutritious diet, and protection from potentially harmful infections and toxins. "At one point we made a commitment as a society to clean up the air and reduce the lead content of our children's teeth, bones, and brains," Dr. Robbins said. "We haven't followed through too well on that, partly because not everyone is convinced that low levels of exposure are dangerous. However, it seems only prudent to me to do all we can to avoid exposing our children, prenatally or after birth, to any toxin."

In addition, Dr. Robbins went on, pregnant women should avoid drugs that are not known to be safe for use during pregnancy (unless the mother has a condition such as epilepsy, so that her need for the drug outweighs the risks involved). "For example," he said, "I personally would be prepared to recommend that a pregnant woman should not have much to drink. Dr. Streissguth, do you agree?"

Dr. Streissguth said there was still a need for more research in this area, but "as a basic public health stance, I would say that it's better for an unborn child not to be exposed to cytomegalovirus, and also better for it not to be exposed to alcohol. I strongly support the Surgeon General's statement recommending that pregnant women not drink."

"It seems clear," Dr. Needleman contributed,

that some remedies now available which could be applied with urgency to groups at high risk would be to feed the brain, to shield it from avoidable toxins, and to give it interesting things to do. If we did that, the number of children who were not doing well at school would be reduced. Learning problems would not disappear, for sure. Then one could deal with the residual number of children with problems of unknown etiology. That's where we desperately need a good nosology, and additional epidemiological and experimental research.

Dr. Needleman added that a better match between teaching and learning style might help in some cases. Dr. Silver suggested, for example, abandoning the usual practice of placing elementary school children in reading groups according to ability. "Instead of three reading groups that all the kids know are good readers, medium readers, and not-so-good readers, you could have one reading group that uses the phonics method, one using the visual method, and one using a multisensorial method. If children could be taught by the method that best fit their individual nervous systems, those with disabilities would have many fewer problems."

Joyce Riley questioned the advisability of an emphasis on classroom remedies. "Even though we assess in the area of neurobiology," she said, "the present treatment of learning disabilities is often pedagogical or educational. It almost seems that the aim is to help the teacher—by training her to deal with distractibility, for instance—instead of to help children function better. If the problem is basically medical, don't we need a medical solution rather than an educational one?"

"I would say we need both," answered Dr. Robbins. "If there's one thing we've learned by sitting down and talking together at this Round Table, it is that different causal factors can have different results. Further, those results can be modified by a variety of events. Some, whether medical or pedagogical, are therapeutically designed, and others are not." With that comment, Dr. Robbins brought the meeting to a close.

GENERAL BIBLIOGRAPHY

Adamsons, K. 1975. Obstetric consideration in the prevention of perinatal asphyxia. In K. Adamsons & H. Fox (Eds.), *Preventability of perinatal injury*. New York: Liss.

Alper, M. H. 1977. Anesthesia and asphyxia. In L. Gluck (Ed.), *Intrauterine asphyxia and the developing fetal brain*. Chicago: Yearbook Medical Publishers.

Balow, B., Rubin, R., & Rosen, M. 1975-1976. Perinatal events as precursors of reading disability. *Reading Research Quarterly* 11:36-71.

Beckwith, L., & Cohen, S. E. In press. Home environment and cognitive competence in preterm children in the first five years. In A. W. Gottfried (Ed.), *Home environment and early mental development*. New York: Academic Press.

Berendes, H. W. 1975. The epidemiology of perinatal injury. In K. Adamsons & H. Fox (Eds.), *Preventability of perinatal injury*. New York: Liss.

Broman, S. H. In press. The Collaborative Perinatal Project: An overview. In S. A. Mednick & M. Harway (Eds.), *Longitudinal research in the United States*. New York: Praeger.

Broman, S. H. 1981. Risk factors for deficits in early cognitive development. In G. G. Berg & H. D. Maillie (Eds.), *Measurement of risks*. New York: Plenum.

Chessex, P., Reichman, B., Verellen, G., Putet, G., Smith, J. M., Heim, T., & Swyer, P. R. 1983. Quality of growth in premature infants fed their own mothers' milk. *Journal of Pediatrics* 102:107-112.

Colletti, L. F. 1979. Relationship between pregnancy and birth complications and the later development of learning disabilities. *Journal of Learning Disabilities* 12:659-663.

Cravioto, J., & Delicardie, E. R. 1979. Nutrition, mental development, and learning. In F. Falkner & J. M. Tanner (Eds.), *Human growth, Vol. 3: Neurobiology and nutrition*. New York: Plenum.

Feder, H. H. 1981. Perinatal hormones and their role in the development of sexually dimorphic behaviors. In N. T. Adler (Ed.), *Neuroendocrinology of reproduction*. New York: Plenum.

Fianu, S., & Joelsson, I. 1979. Minimal brain dysfunction in children born in breech presentation. *Acta Obstetrica Gynecologica Scandinavica* 58:295-299.

Friedman, S. L., & Sigman, M. (Eds.), 1981. *Preterm birth and psychological development*. New York: Academic Press.

Geschwind, N., & Behan, P. 1982. Left-handedness: Association with immune disease, migraine, and developmental learning disorder. *Proceedings of the National Academy of Sciences* 79:5097-5100.

Gibbs, C. E., & Seitchik, J. 1980. Nutrition in pregnancy. In R. S. Goodhart & M. E. Shils (Eds.), *Modern nutrition in health and disease.* Philadelphia: Lea & Febiger.

Graziani, L. J., Mason, J. C., & Cracco, J. 1981. Neurological aspects and early recognition of brain dysfunction in children: Diagnostic and prognostic significance of gestational, perinatal, and postnatal factors. In P. Black (Ed.), *Brain dysfunction in children.* New York: Raven Press.

Haire, D. 1977. The prevention of birth trauma and injury through education for childbearing. In B. L. Blum (Ed.), *Psychological aspects of pregnancy, birthing, and bonding.* New York: Human Sciences Press.

Harvey, D., Prince, J., Bunton, J., Parkinson, C., & Campbell, S. 1982. Abilities of children who were small-for-gestational-age babies. *Pediatrics* 69:296-300.

Hier, D. B. 1979. Sex differences in hemispheric specialization: Hypothesis for the excess of dyslexia in boys. *Bulletin of the Orton Society* 29:74-83.

Hofer, M. A. 1981. Toward a developmental basis for disease predisposition: The effects of early maternal separation on brain, behavior and cardiovascular system. In H. Weiner, M. A. Hofer, & A. J. Stunkard (Eds.), *Brain, behavior and bodily disease.* New York: Raven Press.

Kaffman, M., Sivan-Sher, A., & Carel, C. 1981. Obstetric history of kibbutz children with minimal brain dysfunction. *Israeli Journal of Psychiatry and Related Sciences* 18:69-84.

Kirk, S. A., & Kirk, W. D. 1983. On defining learning disabilities. *Journal of Learning Disabilities* 16:20-21.

Kopp, C. B., & Parmelee, A. H. 1979. Prenatal and perinatal influences on infant behavior. In J. Osofsky (Ed.), *Handbook of Infant Development.* New York: Wiley.

Kraemer, H. C., Korner, A. F., & Thoman, E. B. 1972. Methodological considerations in evaluating the influence of drugs used during labor and delivery on the behavior of the newborn. *Developmental Psychology* 6:128-134.

Levy, H. L., Kaplan, G. N., & Erickson, A. M. 1982. Comparison of treated and untreated pregnancies in a mother with phenylketonuria. *Journal of Pediatrics* 100:876-880.

McEwen, B. S. 1981. Endocrine effects on the brain and their relationship to behavior. In G. Segal et al. (Eds.), *Current topics in neuroendocrinology.* Boston: Little, Brown.

McGlone, J. 1980. Sex differences in human brain asymmetry: A critical survey. *The Behavioral and Brain Sciences* 3:215-263.

Metcoff, J., Costiloe, J. P., Crosby, W., Bentle, L., Seshachalam, D., Sandstead, H. H., Bodwell, C. E., Weaver, F., & McClain, P. 1981. Maternal nutrition and fetal outcome. *American Journal of Clinical Nutrition* 34:708-721 (supplement).

National Research Council. 1976. *Maternal and child health research.* Washington, DC : National Academy of Sciences.

Nichols, P. L., & Chen, T-C. 1981. *Minimal brain dysfunction: A prospective study.* Hillsdale, NJ: Erlbaum.

Oliver, T. K., Jr., Kirschbaum, T. H. (Eds.), & Siegel, L. S. (Guest Ed.). 1982. Low birthweight infants. *Seminars in perinatalogy* 6.

Sameroff, A. J. 1979. The etiology of congnitive competence: A systems perspective. In R. B. Kearsley & I. E. Sigel (Eds.), *Infants at risk: Assessment of cognitive functioning.* Hillsdale, NJ: Erlbaum.

Scanlon, J. W. 1974. Obstetric anesthesia as a neonatal risk factor in normal labor and delivery. *Clinics in perinatology* 1:465-482.

Susser, M. 1981. Prenatal nutrition, birthweight, and psychological development: An overview of experiments, quasi-experiments, and natural experiments in the past decade. *American Journal of Clinical Nutrition* 34:784-803 (supplement).

Waisbren, S. E., Norman, T. R., Schnell, R. R., & Levy, H. L. 1983. Speech and language deficits in early-treated children with galactosemia. *Journal of Pediatrics* 102:75-77.

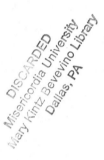